Intermittent Fasting For Women Over 50

Unlock your ageless vitality: 30-day intermittent fasting for women over 50 to rejuvenate your metabolism, shed pounds and ignite energy

Megan Daves

described herein. Additionally, the information in the following pages is intended only for informational purposes and should thus be thought of as universal. As befitting its nature, it is presented without assurance regarding its prolonged validity or interim quality. Trademarks that are mentioned are done without written consent and can in no way be considered an endorsement from the trademark holder.

BONUS: INTERMITTENT FASTING FOR WOMEN OVER 50 – RECIPES

Table of Contents

Introduction

Welcome to Your New Beginning

As the sun rises, casting its first light over the horizon, it brings with it the promise of a new day. So too does your journey into the world of intermittent fasting after 50 usher in a dawn of transformation and renewal. This isn't just a book; it's a gateway to a journey that redefines what it means to age with vitality, grace, and strength. The path you're about to embark on is one filled with discovery, not just about the science of intermittent fasting, but about yourself, your resilience, and your capacity for change.

You stand at the threshold of what can only be described as a new beginning. It's a term often bandied about, yet here it holds a profound truth. The decision to explore intermittent fasting at this stage in your life is not merely about adopting a dietary strategy; it's a bold statement of your willingness to embrace change, to seek out vitality, and to reclaim a sense of control over your health and well-being. This is about more than just shedding pounds or navigating the metabolic shifts that come with age; it's about awakening a zest for life that perhaps you feared was slipping away.

Imagine for a moment the feeling of waking up each morning with more energy than you've had in years, of looking in the mirror and seeing a reflection that radiates health and vitality.

Picture yourself engaging in activities you love, with a body and mind sharpened and sustained by a way of eating that syncs with your body's natural rhythms. This is the promise of intermittent fasting for women over 50, a promise that is as much about renewing your spirit as it is about rejuvenating your body.

But why intermittent fasting, and why now? The beauty of this approach lies in its simplicity and its profound alignment with the ancient wisdom of our bodies. Our ancestors didn't have constant access to food, and their bodies adapted to thrive on periods of fasting and feasting. Today, we find ourselves inundated with the opposite: a constant barrage of meals, snacks, and sugary temptations. This shift has not been kind to our bodies or our metabolic health. Intermittent fasting offers a way back, a way to reset and harmonize with our inherent biological rhythms.

Yet, as you stand on the cusp of this new beginning, it's natural to feel a mix of excitement and apprehension. Change, especially in the context of our dietary habits and lifestyle, can be daunting. You may wonder if it's too late to make a difference, to turn the tide in favor of health and vitality. Let me assure you, it's never too late. The human body is a marvel of adaptability and resilience, capable of remarkable transformation at any age. And intermittent fasting, with its deep roots in our physiological makeup, offers a particularly potent means of tapping into that transformative power.

As we journey through this book together, I invite you to approach it with an open heart and a curious mind. This is an exploration, not just of a dietary pattern, but of what it means to live fully, to age with agency, and to embrace each day with a renewed sense of possibility. It's about finding joy in the simple act of nourishing your body, in discovering the foods and rhythms that make you feel alive, vibrant, and at peace.

This new beginning is also a call to adventure. It's an opportunity to experiment, to learn, and to grow. You'll find that intermittent fasting is as much about the journey as it is about the destination. There will be moments of challenge, of course, but also moments of profound joy and satisfaction. You'll learn to listen to your body in a way you perhaps never have before, to distinguish between true hunger and the myriad other reasons we eat. And in doing so, you'll discover a profound sense of empowerment and autonomy over your health.

So, as you turn these pages and step into the world of intermittent fasting for women over 50, remember that this is your journey. It's uniquely yours, shaped by your experiences, your body, your goals, and your dreams. There's no one "right" way to embark on this path, only your way. And along this journey, you'll find that the true gift of intermittent fasting isn't just the health benefits you'll accrue—it's the deeper connection to yourself, your body, and the world around you.

Welcome, then, to your new beginning. A journey of discovery, transformation, and renewal awaits. Let's embrace this adventure together, with open hearts, curious minds, and the shared goal of unlocking an ageless vitality that shines from within. This is not just the start of a new chapter in your dietary habits; it's the dawn of a new day in your life.

The Power of Intermittent Dieting After 50

As the curtain rises on the second act of life, a time when the wisdom of years begins to interlace with the need for a renewed focus on health, the concept of intermittent dieting emerges not just as a trend but as a beacon of hope. This isn't about dieting in the conventional sense, fraught with restrictions and fleeting results. It's about a transformation that goes beyond the scale, touching the very essence of how we live, age, and thrive. The power of intermittent dieting after 50 is a testament to the strength we harbor within, a strength that only grows with time, ready to be unleashed.

This chapter isn't just a discussion; it's a revelation. It unveils the untapped potential that lies in the rhythm of fasting and feasting, a rhythm as old as time, yet as fresh as the dawn. It's about understanding that after 50, our bodies aren't winding down; they're waiting to be reawakened. The science of intermittent fasting offers not just a key to weight management, but a doorway to a vitality that many thought was lost to the years. It's a vitality that radiates from within, powered by a metabolism reignited, by hormones balanced, and by energy levels that surge like the tides.

Yet, to harness this power, one must first understand the landscape of the body after 50. It's a time of change, yes, but also of immense opportunity. The hormonal shifts and metabolic adjustments that come with age are not obstacles but stepping stones, leading us toward a deeper, more intuitive connection with our health. Intermittent dieting taps into this connection, aligning our eating patterns with our body's natural cycles, promoting healing, and restoration from within. It's a practice that honors our body's wisdom, asking us to listen, really listen, to what it needs.

But what makes intermittent dieting after 50 truly powerful is its flexibility, its ability to mold itself to the individual, to fit into lives full of complexity, history, and beauty. It's not a one-size-fits-all solution but a tapestry of options, each thread woven from the latest research, from ancient practices, and from the stories of those who've walked this path before us. Whether it's the 16/8 method, the 5:2 approach, or any number of variations, the core principle remains the same: balance. Balance between fasting and feasting, between rest and activity, between giving our bodies what they need and allowing them the space to repair and rejuvenate.

In embracing intermittent dieting after 50, we also embrace a shift in perspective. It's a move away from viewing food as merely fuel or even as a foe in the battle of the bulge. Instead, food becomes a partner in our journey, a source of nourishment, joy, and celebration. This perspective shift is crucial, for it's not just our bodies that benefit from intermittent fasting; our minds and spirits are uplifted as well. The clarity of thought, the surge in creativity, the deep, restorative sleep—these are but a few of the gifts that come with this way of life.

Yet, amidst the science and the stories, there lies a simple truth: the power of intermittent dieting after 50 is not just in the physiological benefits, but in the rediscovery of ourselves. It's a journey that challenges us to break free from the myths of aging, to redefine what it means to grow older. It's about finding strength in the softness, resilience in the rest, and beauty in the balance. This way of eating, this way of living, becomes a canvas on which we paint our second act, vibrant and full of life.

As you stand at the precipice of this new beginning, know that the power of intermittent dieting after 50 is within your grasp. It's a power that comes from knowledge, from understanding, and from the courage to embrace change. This chapter, this book, is your companion on the journey, a guide to unlocking the vitality that awaits. It's an invitation to live fully, to age gracefully, and to meet the coming years with a spirit undimmed by time.

In this exploration of intermittent dieting, remember that the true power lies not in the fasting itself, but in the reawakening it brings. It's a reawakening of the body, certainly, but also of the heart and mind. It's a testament to the enduring strength and adaptability that defines us, a reminder that after 50, life is not just to be lived—it's to be celebrated, with every fast broken and every feast savored.

Navigating This Book for Maximum Benefit

Embarking on the journey through the pages of this book is akin to setting sail on a grand voyage across uncharted waters. The destination is a land where vitality and wellness reign supreme, and the compass guiding you is the knowledge and wisdom contained within these chapters. As you navigate through "Navigating This Book for Maximum Benefit," consider this section your map, your North Star, guiding you to extract the richest treasures from our collective exploration of intermittent fasting for women over 50.

This book is more than a collection of facts and guidelines; it is a tapestry woven from the threads of science, personal stories, and practical advice, designed to guide you through the complexities of intermittent fasting with ease and clarity. To fully embrace the transformative power of this journey, it's essential to approach this book not as a passive reader but as an active participant in your own story of renewal and discovery.

Imagine, if you will, a garden. Just as a gardener tills the soil, plants the seeds, and nurtures the growth, so too will you cultivate your understanding, sow the practices of intermittent fasting, and foster a lifestyle of health and vitality. Each chapter, each section, is a stepping stone on this path, leading you toward a deeper connection with your body, a harmonious relationship with food, and a vibrant, energized existence.

The structure of this book is intentionally designed to guide you through the layers of understanding and application, from the foundational principles of intermittent fasting to the nuanced strategies for integrating it into your life. It begins with the soil—the essential knowledge about your body after 50, the metabolic and hormonal shifts, and the science behind aging and weight. This foundational knowledge serves as the bedrock upon which your intermittent fasting journey will be built.

As we delve deeper, we explore the seeds of practice—the various intermittent fasting plans and how to choose the one that resonates with your body's unique needs and your lifestyle. This section is not about prescribing a one-size-fits-all solution but about empowering you to make informed choices that align with your goals, your health, and your joy.

Watering and nurturing your garden comes next, with chapters dedicated to mindset and motivation, the integration of movement, and the art of nutrition and cooking for vitality.

These sections are your guide to cultivating a positive outlook, setting achievable goals, and embracing physical activity and nourishing foods as sources of pleasure and strength.

But a garden is more than just soil, seeds, and water; it's a living ecosystem, rich in diversity and interconnectedness. Similarly, this book acknowledges the ecosystem of your life— your routines, your relationships, your joys, and your challenges. It offers strategies for weaving intermittent fasting into the fabric of your daily existence, ensuring that it enriches your life rather than complicates it.

In navigating this book for maximum benefit, remember that your journey is unique. While the chapters are laid out in a manner that builds understanding and application step by step, feel free to approach them in a way that best suits your curiosity and needs. You might find yourself drawn to the chapters on mindset and motivation early on, seeking the inspiration to embark on this path. Or perhaps the practical aspects of meal planning and exercise resonate more strongly at the outset. Trust your intuition; it is a powerful guide on this journey.

Throughout this voyage, be patient with yourself. Just as a garden doesn't bloom overnight, the benefits of intermittent fasting unfold over time. Celebrate the small victories, the subtle shifts in energy and well-being, and the deeper understanding of your body and its needs. These are the true markers of progress, the signs that you are moving ever closer to your destination of health, vitality, and a life lived fully and joyously.

In essence, navigating this book for maximum benefit is about embracing the journey with an open heart and a curious mind. It's about finding your rhythm, listening to your body, and allowing the principles of intermittent fasting to weave their way into your life in a manner that feels nourishing, sustainable, and joyful.

Part I: Understanding Your Body After 50

The Metabolic Shift: Embracing Change

Hormonal Harmony: Menopause and Metabolism

Navigating through the later chapters of life, especially after crossing the threshold of 50, presents a tapestry of changes, challenges, and opportunities. Among the most pivotal of these shifts is the transformation that occurs within our metabolic and hormonal landscapes. This narrative journey into "Hormonal Harmony: Menopause and Metabolism" seeks to unravel the complexities of this transition, illuminating paths towards understanding, acceptance, and strategic adaptation.

As the curtain rises on this chapter of life, many women find themselves at a crossroads, where the physical and emotional changes brought on by menopause intersect with evolving metabolic rates. This period, often marked by fluctuating hormones, heralds a time of profound change, impacting everything from energy levels to weight management. Yet, within this flux lies an opportunity—an invitation to embrace these changes with knowledge, grace, and empowered action.

Menopause, a natural biological process, signifies the end of menstrual cycles, a milestone typically occurring in a woman's 40s or 50s. It's defined by a significant hormonal shift, primarily involving decreased production of estrogen and progesterone. These hormones, beyond their role in reproduction, exert a powerful influence on metabolism—the complex biochemical process by which our bodies convert food into energy.

The interplay between these hormonal adjustments and metabolism is intricate. Estrogen, for instance, helps regulate body weight and energy expenditure. With its decline, women often experience a reduction in metabolic rate, making it easier to gain weight, especially around the abdomen. This shift is not merely cosmetic; it carries implications for cardiovascular health, bone density, and overall well-being.

However, understanding this transition offers more than just insight into why these changes occur; it provides a foundation upon which to build strategies for health and vitality. The first step is recognizing the role of muscle mass. As we age, muscle naturally diminishes, a process known as sarcopenia, which can slow metabolism further. Yet, this is not an inevitable decline into inactivity. Resistance training and protein-rich diets can counteract these effects, preserving muscle mass and, by extension, metabolic rate.

Dietary considerations play a crucial role as well. The nutritional needs of our bodies evolve over time, demanding a closer examination of what we eat, how much, and when. This is where the concept of intermittent fasting enters the conversation—not as a trend, but as a tool for metabolic reawakening. By alternating periods of eating with fasting, intermittent fasting can stimulate metabolic flexibility, encouraging the body to shift more efficiently between energy sources.

Intermittent fasting also dovetails with the hormonal milieu of menopause. It can improve insulin sensitivity, a boon given the increased risk of insulin resistance during this period. Moreover, the practice has been linked to improvements in markers of inflammation and oxidative stress, both of which are pivotal in navigating menopause with health and grace.

Yet, the journey through menopause is as personal as it is physiological. It's a narrative woven from individual experiences, health histories, and personal goals. This underscores the importance of a tailored approach—one that considers not only the biological underpinnings of menopause and metabolism but also the unique lifestyle, preferences, and challenges of each woman.

Embracing change, therefore, becomes a multifaceted endeavor. It's about nurturing the body with movement and mindful nutrition, certainly. But it's also about fostering emotional well-being, seeking support, and cultivating resilience. This chapter of life, with all its nuances, is not merely one to be endured but to be lived fully, with intention and joy.

In navigating the metabolic shift brought on by menopause, knowledge is power. Understanding the biological currents that shape this transition can demystify the experience, transforming it from a source of frustration into an opportunity for growth and health. Armed with this knowledge, women can approach their 50s and beyond not with trepidation but with confidence, equipped to make informed choices that support their well-being in this new chapter of life.

The Science of Aging and Weight

As we journey through the chapters of our lives, the narrative of our bodies undergoes its own profound evolution, especially as we cross the threshold of 50. This pivotal stage marks not just a chronological milestone but a transformation in the very essence of how we interact with the world around us, particularly in terms of our metabolism and weight. "The Science of Aging and Weight" is not merely a chapter in a book; it is a window into understanding the intricate ballet of biological processes that define aging and its impact on our body's ability to manage weight.

Embarking on this exploration requires a departure from the beaten path of conventional wisdom. It demands that we delve deeper into the cellular level, where the secrets of aging are whispered among the mitochondria, the DNA, and the proteins that orchestrate our existence. Aging, as it turns out, is not just a linear progression but a complex adaptive process that reflects the cumulative impact of time on our cells and systems.

At the heart of this process is metabolism, the alchemical laboratory within our bodies that transforms food into energy. This metabolic rate, often taken for granted during the flush of youth, begins to decelerate with age. This deceleration is a symphony of factors, including the gradual loss of muscle mass, hormonal adjustments, and changes in cellular efficiency. Muscle, a voracious consumer of calories, dwindles in a process known as sarcopenia, diminishing our metabolic baseline and making weight gain more likely and weight loss more challenging.

But the plot thickens when we consider the role of hormones in this narrative. Hormones, those biochemical messengers that carry whispers and commands across the body, also shift with age. Insulin, for example, becomes less effective at ushering glucose into cells, a change that can nudge the body toward insulin resistance and contribute to weight gain. Similarly, changes in sex hormones like estrogen and testosterone have their own roles to play in the story of aging and weight.

Yet, understanding these changes offers not just insight but empowerment. It reveals that aging and weight management are not merely about calories in versus calories out but about understanding and adapting to the changes within our bodies. It invites a more nuanced approach to nutrition, one that respects the body's evolving needs for protein, vitamins, minerals, and other nutrients to support muscle mass, bone density, and overall vitality.

This chapter also illuminates the often-overlooked role of lifestyle factors in navigating the metabolic shifts of aging. Sleep, often the first casualty in our busy lives, emerges as a critical player in metabolic health. Quality sleep acts as a reset button for metabolism, supporting hormonal balance, appetite regulation, and insulin sensitivity. Stress, too, takes center stage, with its ability to disrupt hormonal equilibrium and encourage the storage of abdominal fat through the action of cortisol.

In this light, the journey of aging becomes a call to action—a prompt to embrace lifestyle choices that support metabolic health, from prioritizing sleep and managing stress to engaging in regular physical activity that builds muscle and enhances flexibility.

But perhaps the most empowering aspect of understanding the science of aging and weight is the realization that we are not powerless in the face of time. While we may not be able to turn back the clock, we can influence how our bodies navigate the passage of years. This understanding paves the way for strategies like intermittent fasting, which we will explore in depth in the coming chapters. Intermittent fasting offers a promising approach to recalibrating our metabolic machinery, optimizing hormonal balance, and embracing the aging process with grace, vitality, and a sense of control.

Intermittent Fasting: Is It Right for You?

Intermittent fasting (IF) is not just a dietary trend but a lens through which we can reimagine our relationship with food, our bodies, and the rhythm of our daily lives. As we venture beyond the half-century mark, the quest for vitality and health takes on new dimensions. The metabolic and hormonal shifts that accompany this era of life beckon for a nuanced approach to nutrition—one that honors our body's changing needs and harnesses the power of timing to rejuvenate and heal. Intermittent fasting emerges as a beacon in this journey, offering a path that diverges from traditional diets to focus on when we eat as much as what we eat.

At its core, intermittent fasting involves cycling between periods of eating and fasting. It's a practice rooted in the rhythms of nature and our evolutionary history, echoing the feast and famine cycles our ancestors navigated. This rhythm, some argue, is one our bodies inherently understand and thrive on. But the question looms large: Is intermittent fasting the right choice for you, especially after the age of 50?

To answer this, we must first delve into the science that

underpins intermittent fasting, exploring how it interacts with our bodies at a cellular level. Research suggests that IF can influence numerous biological pathways that are pivotal as we age. It can enhance autophagy, the process by which our cells cleanse themselves of damaged components, thereby promoting cellular repair and renewal. It can also improve insulin sensitivity, reduce inflammation, and potentially support cognitive function by encouraging the production of brain-derived neurotrophic factor (BDNF).

Moreover, intermittent fasting's impact on hormonal balance is of particular interest during the post-menopausal years. The hormonal ebbs and flows of menopause can complicate metabolic health, making weight management a challenge for many women. IF offers a tool to potentially recalibrate this balance, leveraging periods of fasting to stabilize insulin levels and moderate the body's fat storage mechanisms.

Yet, the decision to embrace intermittent fasting is deeply personal and should be approached with consideration of one's individual health history, lifestyle, and wellness goals. It's a practice that requires tuning in to the body's signals, recognizing the difference between beneficial stress and undue strain. For some, the structured eating windows of IF can foster a renewed sense of dietary freedom and control, simplifying meal planning and reducing the constant decision-making associated with traditional diets. For others, the adjustment to fasting periods can be challenging, particularly if underlying health issues, such as diabetes or hypoglycemia, are present.

Thus, embarking on an intermittent fasting journey after 50 is as much about introspection as it is about nutrition. It involves assessing not just your dietary preferences and lifestyle, but also engaging with healthcare professionals to ensure that your approach to IF aligns with your overall health objectives and medical needs. It's about considering how fasting fits into your daily routine, your social life, and your personal relationship with food.

The beauty of intermittent fasting lies in its flexibility. There are various approaches to IF, from the 16/8 method, where eating is confined to an 8-hour window, to 5:2 strategies, which involve normal eating for five days and reduced calorie intake for two. This flexibility allows for personalization, enabling individuals to experiment and find the rhythm that feels most sustainable and beneficial for them.

As we navigate the narrative of our lives, the chapters post-50 offer a unique opportunity to redefine health and well-being on our terms. Intermittent fasting, with its blend of ancient wisdom and modern science, invites us to explore a different path—one that emphasizes the timing of nourishment as a key to unlocking vitality. It's a journey of discovery, requiring an open mind, a willing spirit, and a commitment to listening deeply to the wisdom of our bodies.

In conclusion, "Intermittent Fasting: Is It Right for You?" is not just a question; it's an invitation. An invitation to explore, to experiment, and to engage with our health in a proactive and empowered way. As with any journey, there are considerations and cautions, but for many, the path of intermittent fasting after 50 offers a promising route to rejuvenation, vitality, and a deepened connection to the rhythms of our bodies and our lives.

Decoding Hunger: Insights Into Appetite Control

The Role of Ghrelin and Leptin

In the intricate dance of life after 50, understanding the body's signals becomes paramount, especially when it comes to hunger and satiety. The quest for balance in appetite control is a nuanced journey, deeply influenced by two key players: ghrelin and leptin. These hormones, far from being mere biological footnotes, are the conductors of our body's symphony, orchestrating the ebb and flow of hunger and fullness. Deciphering their roles offers a gateway to harmonizing our relationship with food, a relationship that often becomes complicated as we age.

Ghrelin, known colloquially as the "hunger hormone," is produced in the stomach and signals the brain to stimulate appetite. Its levels rise when the stomach is empty and decrease after eating. Picture ghrelin as a messenger, briskly traveling through the body, announcing the need to replenish energy. In an ideal world, ghrelin's message is clear and timely, guiding us to eat when our body truly needs nourishment. However, as we cross the threshold of 50, the clarity of this message can become muddled, influenced by factors such as stress, sleep deprivation, and changes in body composition.

Leptin, on the other hand, is the "satiety hormone," primarily produced by fat cells. It communicates with the brain to signal fullness, telling us to put down the fork. Leptin's role is to maintain energy balance, to prevent overeating and promote energy expenditure. Yet, the plot thickens with the introduction of leptin resistance, a condition where the body, despite having ample fat stores (and thus high levels of leptin), becomes less sensitive to its signals. This resistance can create a paradoxical state where, despite being physically full, the brain perceives hunger, leading to overeating.

The interplay between ghrelin and leptin is a delicate balance, one that is essential for maintaining healthy weight and energy levels. However, this balance can be disrupted by the hormonal changes and lifestyle shifts that accompany aging. For instance, reduced physical activity and muscle mass can alter the body's response to these hormones, as can changes in sleep patterns and stress levels.

Understanding this hormonal tango is the first step in

mastering appetite control after 50. It's about listening to the body's cues, discerning true hunger from habit, and responding with mindfulness and intention. This knowledge empowers us to navigate the changing landscape of our bodies with grace, making informed choices that support our health and well-being.

But knowledge alone is not enough. It must be coupled with practical strategies for tuning into ghrelin and leptin's signals and responding appropriately. This is where the principles of mindful eating come into play, inviting us to eat with awareness and appreciation, to savor each bite, and to listen to our body's cues of hunger and fullness. Mindful eating encourages us to pause before reaching for food, to consider whether we're truly hungry or if we're seeking to feed an emotional need.

Moreover, understanding ghrelin and leptin can also inform our approach to meal timing and composition. Eating balanced meals with a mix of protein, fiber, and healthy fats can help regulate these hormones, promoting a sense of fullness and reducing the likelihood of overeating. Similarly, establishing a regular eating schedule can help normalize ghrelin levels, preventing the sharp spikes and dips that lead to hunger pangs and cravings.

"The Role of Ghrelin and Leptin" is not just a chapter in the story of appetite control; it's a foundational piece in the larger narrative of aging well. By decoding the messages of these hormones, we unlock the secrets to navigating hunger and fullness with wisdom and ease. This knowledge, combined with mindful practices and a balanced approach to nutrition, allows us to cultivate a relationship with food that nourishes not just our bodies but our souls.

Thus, as we journey through the later chapters of life, let us embrace the wisdom that comes with age, including the insights into our body's inner workings. Let ghrelin and leptin be our guides, leading us to a place of balance and harmony in our relationship with food, a place where every meal is an opportunity for nourishment, pleasure, and gratitude.

Mindful Eating Practices

Embarking on the journey of mindful eating practices is akin to entering a sanctuary where each meal becomes a meditation, a moment of connection between body, mind, and the earth that provides our nourishment. In a world where eating often becomes an automated task performed alongside other activities, mindful eating invites us to pause, to breathe, and to truly engage with the act of nourishing ourselves. This practice, especially for those navigating the nuances of life after 50, becomes a cornerstone of understanding and controlling appetite, transforming the act of eating from a mere biological necessity into a profound ritual of self-care and awareness.

Mindful eating is not about strict diets or deprivation but about fostering a deep, intuitive relationship with food. It starts with listening—really listening—to our body's signals of hunger and fullness, distinguishing between the physiological need to eat and the myriad other reasons we might feel drawn to food, be it boredom, stress, or emotional comfort. This attentiveness to our body's cues requires a shift away from the distractions that often accompany meals, encouraging us to eat without the accompaniment of screens, books, or stressful conversations. By doing so, we allow ourselves the space to notice the flavors, textures, and aromas of our food, to appreciate the way it looks on the plate, and to honor the journey it took to reach our table.

The practice of mindful eating also invites us to explore our food preferences and aversions with curiosity rather than judgment, to experiment with new flavors and textures, and to notice how different foods affect our energy, mood, and overall well-being. This exploration is particularly poignant in the later chapters of life, where nutritional needs shift and the metabolism slows, making it even more essential to choose foods that nourish and satiate us deeply.

Mindful eating also encompasses the preparation of food, turning the act of cooking into a mindful practice in itself. It encourages us to engage with the process of creating meals, from selecting ingredients to chopping and cooking them, as an act of self-love and care. This approach to food preparation not only deepens our connection with what we eat but also allows us to imbue our meals with intention and gratitude, qualities that enhance the nourishing properties of food.

Moreover, mindful eating challenges the cultural narratives around aging and appetite, narratives that often frame the later years as a time of inevitable decline and limitation. Instead, it presents an opportunity to reframe our relationship with food as we age, seeing this time as an invitation to deepen our understanding of our bodies and to nourish them with the respect and care they deserve. By doing so, we not only support our physical health but also cultivate a sense of abundance and joy in our eating experiences.

In practice, mindful eating involves simple, accessible habits that can transform our meals: eating slowly and without distraction, tuning into the sensations of taste and texture, pausing mid-meal to assess our fullness, and approaching our meals with gratitude. These practices help to recalibrate our appetite control, making us more attuned to our body's needs and less likely to overeat or indulge in foods that don't serve our well-being.

At its heart, mindful eating is a journey back to ourselves, a way to reclaim the act of eating as a sacred, nourishing practice that supports our health, happiness, and overall quality of life. It's an invitation to savor each bite, to listen deeply to our bodies, and to eat with intention and joy. As we navigate the changing landscape of our bodies and lives after

50, mindful eating becomes not just a strategy for appetite control, but a pathway to a more connected, conscious, and fulfilling way of living.

Overcoming Cravings and Emotional Eating

In the rich tapestry of life after 50, navigating the complex world of cravings and emotional eating emerges as a pivotal chapter in our journey towards health and harmony. This stage of life brings its own unique set of challenges and transitions, from changes in metabolism to shifts in lifestyle and identity, all of which can profoundly influence our relationship with food. Overcoming cravings and emotional eating isn't just about willpower; it's about understanding the underlying narratives that drive these behaviors and rewiring our responses to food to nourish both body and soul.

Cravings and emotional eating often serve as a language through which our body communicates deeper needs—needs that may not be solely about hunger but about seeking comfort, alleviating stress, or numbing emotions. Recognizing this language requires a gentle, introspective approach, one that invites us to pause and ask, "What am I really hungry for?" This question is not a mere rhetorical flourish but a tool for self-discovery, opening a dialogue with ourselves about our needs, desires, and the ways in which we seek fulfillment.

As we embark on this exploration, it becomes clear that

cravings are not the enemy but signals, guiding us towards a deeper understanding of our emotional landscape. They beckon us to explore not just the foods we crave but the emotions and situations that trigger these cravings. Is it loneliness, boredom, stress, or sadness that sends us in search of comfort in the pantry? By mapping these triggers, we create a blueprint for navigating our cravings with awareness and compassion.

Transforming our relationship with emotional eating requires cultivating a repertoire of strategies that support our well-being beyond the momentary satisfaction of indulging a craving. This toolkit includes practices like mindful breathing, which can help center and calm us, reducing the immediacy of the craving. It encompasses finding alternative sources of comfort and fulfillment, such as engaging in a hobby, connecting with a friend, or immersing oneself in nature, activities that nourish us without the need for food as a mediator.

Equally important is creating an environment that supports our journey. This involves stocking our kitchens with foods that nourish and satisfy, preparing meals that delight the senses and satiate the body, and cultivating a mindful eating environment where meals are consumed with intention and gratitude, not as a backdrop to other activities. It's about learning to enjoy food for its own sake, savoring flavors, textures, and the act of eating itself, without using food as a means to an emotional end.

Yet, overcoming cravings and emotional eating is not about perfection but about progress, about learning and growing from each experience. It's about developing resilience, the ability to navigate setbacks with grace and to see them not as failures but as opportunities for insight and growth. This journey is deeply personal, one that intertwines the physical, emotional, and spiritual, and it invites us to forge a relationship with food that is based on nourishment, joy, and a profound respect for our bodies and their wisdom.

In this narrative of overcoming cravings and emotional eating, we find not just strategies for managing our appetites but pathways to a richer, more connected life. This chapter is an invitation to explore the depths of our relationship with food, to confront and embrace our vulnerabilities, and to emerge empowered, with a newfound understanding of how to nourish ourselves in every sense of the word. It's a testament to the strength and resilience that come with age, to the capacity for renewal and transformation that defines the human spirit.

Part II: Intermittent Dieting Fundamentals

Blueprint for Success: Choosing Your IF Plan

Evaluating Popular IF Windows: 16/8, 5:2, and More

The 16/8 method, often hailed as the gateway to intermittent fasting, proposes an eating window of 8 hours followed by 16 hours of fasting. This approach, celebrated for its simplicity and adaptability, aligns with the body's natural circadian rhythm, offering a gentle introduction to the world of IF. Imagine, if you will, the ease of skipping breakfast, making your first meal at noon, and completing your evening meal by 8 p.m. This rhythm, for many, fits seamlessly into the fabric of daily life, enhancing metabolic flexibility without the weight of drastic lifestyle changes.

Yet, the journey doesn't end here. The 5:2 method unfolds a different path, one where normal eating patterns are followed for five days a week, punctuated by two days of reduced calorie intake (typically around 500-600 calories per day). This pattern encourages a deeper dive into the fasting experience, challenging the body to adapt to intermittent periods of significant calorie reduction. It's a testament to the body's resilience and adaptability, offering a unique perspective on hunger and satiety.

Beyond these shores lie more nuanced IF approaches, such as the Eat-Stop-Eat method, which involves a 24-hour fast once or twice a week, or the alternate-day fasting, where the rhythm of fasting and eating ebbs and flows with the days of the week. Each of these methods opens a new chapter in the story of IF, inviting individuals to discover the rhythms that resonate most deeply with their personal health narratives.

Choosing the right IF window is not merely a matter of preference; it's a decision grounded in self-awareness and mindful consideration of one's health goals, lifestyle, and the body's signals. It requires tuning into the subtle cues of energy, hunger, and satiety that the body communicates daily. It's about recognizing the difference between the mind's cravings and the body's needs, about finding balance in the ebb and flow of fasting and feasting.

Personalizing your intermittent diet is akin to customizing a suit—it should fit your body's needs, lifestyle demands, and personal goals with precision. This customization might involve starting with a less restrictive fasting approach, such as the 12-hour fast, and gradually extending the fasting window as the body adapts. It's about listening to your body, adjusting the fasting window to accommodate physical activity levels, work schedules, and social engagements, ensuring that IF enhances your life rather than complicating it.

Synchronizing IF with your lifestyle means integrating fasting into your daily life in a way that feels almost seamless. It's about making IF a harmonious part of your routine, not a disruptive force. This integration involves practical considerations, such as planning your fasting windows around social events or work commitments, and emotional ones, like ensuring your fasting practice supports your mental and emotional well-being.

The journey of choosing your IF plan is not a one-size-fits-all voyage. It's a personal exploration, a journey of discovering what works best for your body and your life. It's about navigating through the different fasting windows, experimenting with what feels right, and adjusting course as needed. It's a process that calls for patience, curiosity, and a gentle, forgiving attitude towards oneself.

In the grand tapestry of intermittent fasting, each fasting window, from the 16/8 to the more extended periods of fasting, offers a unique set of benefits and challenges. The key to unlocking these benefits lies not just in the method chosen but in the approach to the journey—embracing IF with openness, adaptability, and a deep commitment to listening to one's body and respecting its needs.

Thus, the blueprint for success in intermittent fasting is not found in rigid adherence to a specific plan but in the fluid, flexible approach to integrating fasting into your life. It's about charting a course that respects your body's signals, aligns with your lifestyle, and moves you towards your health goals with grace and ease. It's a journey that, when navigated thoughtfully, leads not just to a destination of improved physical health, but to a place of deeper self-understanding and harmony.

Personalizing Your Intermittent Diet

The cornerstone of personalizing your intermittent diet lies in the recognition that we are all architects of our own health. Just as a skilled architect draws up plans that reflect both the landscape and the desires of those who will inhabit the space, so too must we design our IF plans with an acute awareness of our physical landscape and our personal and professional commitments. This approach transcends the one-size-fits-all diets that dominate the landscape of nutritional advice, offering instead a bespoke path that honors our individuality.

The first step in this customization process involves a deep dive into self-awareness. Understanding your body's signals, from hunger cues to energy levels throughout the day, provides invaluable insights into the fasting window that might suit you best. Are you a morning person, brimming with energy and barely thinking about food until later in the day? Or do you find your hunger peaks in the morning, suggesting that an eating window that starts earlier might be more in harmony with your natural inclinations?

Equally important is the consideration of your lifestyle and daily routine. For those with a 9-to-5 job, social commitments, or family responsibilities, the flexibility of the fasting schedule is paramount. The beauty of IF lies in its adaptability; whether it's adjusting the eating window to align with family dinners or choosing a fasting day when you're less socially active, the goal is to weave IF seamlessly into the fabric of your life, not to let it stand as an obstacle to living fully.

Moreover, personalizing your IF plan involves tuning into your body's nutritional needs and how they might change during fasting periods. Engaging with a healthcare provider or a nutritionist can provide a solid foundation of knowledge on which to build your IF schedule, ensuring that your dietary choices support your overall health, energy levels, and nutritional requirements. This personalized approach not only maximizes the benefits of IF but also turns it into a sustainable, long-term practice.

Another critical aspect of personalizing your intermittent diet is the willingness to experiment and adjust. The journey of IF is one of discovery, where initial plans may evolve as you gain insights into what works best for your body and lifestyle. This iterative process, grounded in patience and self-compassion, is essential for finding the balance that promotes well-being while also achieving your health goals.

Finally, personalizing your IF plan is about more than just

when you eat; it's about what you eat. Integrating whole, nutrient-dense foods into your eating windows enriches the IF experience, ensuring that your body is nourished and satisfied, making the fasting periods more manageable and more effective. This mindful approach to nutrition complements the physical benefits of fasting with the holistic nourishment of the body and mind.

In essence, personalizing your intermittent diet is a journey of self-discovery, a process that honors your uniqueness and seeks to integrate IF into your life in a way that feels natural, joyful, and sustainable. It's about listening deeply to your body, embracing flexibility, and making informed choices that support your health and happiness. As you navigate this path, remember that the ultimate goal is not just to adapt to IF but to adapt IF to you, crafting a lifestyle that resonates with your body's needs and your life's rhythms. This journey, while deeply personal, is also universally empowering, offering each of us the tools to become the healthiest, most vibrant versions of ourselves. At the heart of personalizing your intermittent diet is the recognition of our roles as architects of our own health. Much like a skilled architect who meticulously designs plans that mirror the landscape's contours and the inhabitants' desires, we, too, must thoughtfully construct our IF plans. This construction requires an acute awareness of our physical and emotional landscapes along with our personal and professional commitments. This strategy moves beyond the generic, one-size-fits-all diets that saturate the nutritional advice landscape, offering, instead, a tailored pathway that celebrates our individuality.

The initial step in this bespoke process demands a deep dive into self-awareness. Tuning into your body's signals—from hunger cues to fluctuations in energy levels throughout the day—yields critical insights into the fasting window that aligns best with your physiological needs. Consider whether you are a morning person, pulsing with energy and scarcely thinking about food until later in the day, or if you find your hunger peaking in the morning, hinting that an eating window commencing earlier may better harmonize with your natural rhythms.

Equally pivotal is the reflection on your lifestyle and daily routines. For individuals juggling a 9-to-5 job, navigating social commitments, or managing family responsibilities, the adaptability of the fasting schedule is paramount. The true beauty of IF lies in its remarkable flexibility; it's about adjusting the eating window to accommodate family meals or selecting fasting days that align with quieter moments in your social calendar. The objective is to weave IF seamlessly into the fabric of your existence, ensuring it complements rather than complicates your way of life.

Furthermore, tailoring your IF plan necessitates an attunement to your body's evolving nutritional needs, particularly during fasting periods. Collaborating with healthcare providers or nutritionists can lay a robust foundation of knowledge, enabling you to construct an IF schedule that bolsters your overall health, vitality, and nutritional well-being. This personalized approach not only elevates the efficacy of IF but also transforms it into a sustainable, enduring practice.

A critical dimension of personalizing your intermittent diet is the openness to experimentation and adjustment. The IF journey is characterized by discovery, where initial plans are often refined as you unearth what resonates best with your body and lifestyle. This evolutionary process, rooted in patience and self-compassion, is crucial for striking a balance that fosters well-being while facilitating the achievement of your health objectives.

Moreover, personalizing your IF regimen encompasses more than the timing of meals; it extends to the quality and substance of what you consume. Incorporating whole, nutrient-rich foods into your eating windows not only enriches the IF experience but also ensures your body is thoroughly nourished and satisfied, rendering fasting periods more manageable and efficacious. This mindful approach to nutrition beautifully complements the physical benefits of fasting, offering holistic nourishment for both body and soul.

Synchronizing IF with Your Lifestyle

Synchronizing intermittent fasting (IF) with your lifestyle is akin to composing a symphony where each element, from the quietest note to the most vibrant crescendo, harmonizes perfectly with your daily rhythms, commitments, and personal aspirations. This alignment is not merely about imposing a fasting regimen onto an existing schedule but rather about weaving IF into the fabric of your life so seamlessly that it amplifies your well-being, energy, and fulfillment. Achieving this synchronization requires a nuanced understanding of your own life's patterns, an openness to adapt and refine, and a commitment to prioritizing your health in a way that feels both rewarding and sustainable.

The first step towards integrating IF into your lifestyle involves a deep dive into the natural ebb and flow of your daily activities and energy levels. Each person's day is punctuated by peaks and troughs of energy, periods of focus, and moments of relaxation. Observing these patterns provides critical insights that can guide the selection of an IF window. For instance, if mornings are your most productive times, starting your day with a nourishing meal might enhance your focus and productivity, suggesting that a later fasting window could be more in tune with your natural rhythm. Conversely, if evenings are when you unwind and enjoy socializing over meals, an earlier eating window that accommodates these activities might be preferable.

A key aspect of synchronizing IF with your lifestyle is embracing flexibility. Life is inherently dynamic, filled with unexpected demands, special occasions, and shifts in routine. A rigid approach to IF can not only create stress but also detract from the enjoyment and benefits of fasting. Instead, adopting a flexible mindset allows you to adjust your fasting windows as needed, accommodating changes without guilt or frustration. This adaptability ensures that IF enhances your life, providing structure without confinement, and supports your well-being without becoming a source of stress.

Aligning IF with both personal and professional commitments is crucial for its long-term sustainability. In the professional realm, consider your work schedule, meetings, and business lunches. Integrating IF might mean adjusting your eating window to ensure you can participate fully in work-related dining without compromising your fasting goals. On the personal front, family meals, social gatherings, and leisure activities all play a significant role in how you structure your fasting. The goal is to find a balance that allows you to honor your commitments to others and yourself, ensuring that IF supports your relationships and personal life rather than hindering them.

Synchronizing IF with your lifestyle also involves a keen focus on health and nutrition. Fasting periods are opportunities to tune into your body's needs, while eating windows present chances to nourish your body with high-quality, nutrient-dense foods. Aligning your IF practice with your nutritional needs means choosing foods that sustain your energy, support your health goals, and satisfy your palate. It also means being mindful of hydration and supplementing your diet as necessary to ensure you're receiving a full spectrum of nutrients.

A harmonious integration of IF into your lifestyle is as much about mindset as it is about mechanics. Approaching IF with curiosity, patience, and self-compassion facilitates a smoother adaptation process. It involves setting realistic expectations, celebrating progress, and viewing setbacks as opportunities for learning and adjustment. Cultivating a positive mindset towards fasting can transform it from a mere dietary strategy into a powerful tool for self-care and personal growth.

Finally, synchronizing IF with your lifestyle is an ongoing process of learning and adjustment. It requires regular reflection on what's working and what isn't, openness to trying new approaches, and the wisdom to make changes that better align with your evolving life and goals. This continuous refinement ensures that your IF practice remains dynamic, responsive, and aligned with your journey towards optimal health and vitality.

In essence, synchronizing intermittent fasting with your lifestyle is about crafting a unique and personal IF symphony, one that resonates with the rhythms of your daily life, enhances your well-being, and supports your journey towards becoming the healthiest, most vibrant version of yourself. It's a deeply personal process that honors your individuality, respects your commitments, and enriches your life, making intermittent fasting a seamlessly integrated aspect of your journey towards health and fulfillment.

The Synergy of Diet and Hormones

Balancing Insulin and Blood Sugar Levels

In the nuanced symphony of the body's metabolic processes, the harmonious interaction between diet and hormones plays a pivotal role, with insulin and blood sugar levels taking center stage. This delicate balance is not just a biological dance of molecules; it's the cornerstone of our well-being, influencing everything from our energy levels to our body's ability to manage weight. The journey to understand and optimize this balance is akin to navigating a complex labyrinth, where each turn represents a choice in diet and lifestyle that can lead us closer to or further from metabolic harmony.

Insulin, a hormone produced by the pancreas, serves as a key player in the regulation of blood sugar levels. Its primary role is to facilitate the uptake of glucose (sugar) from the bloodstream into the cells, where it's used for energy. However, the modern diet, rich in processed foods, sugars, and refined carbohydrates, can lead to spikes in blood sugar levels, prompting the pancreas to release more insulin. Over time, this can lead to insulin resistance, a condition where the cells become less responsive to insulin's signals. This not only elevates blood sugar levels but also disrupts the body's metabolic balance, setting the stage for a host of health issues, including type 2 diabetes and obesity.

Navigating the maze of dietary choices to find those that support insulin sensitivity and blood sugar balance requires both knowledge and intuition. Foods high in fiber, such as vegetables, whole grains, and legumes, play a crucial role in this balance. Fiber slows the absorption of sugar into the bloodstream, helping to prevent the rapid spikes in blood sugar and insulin levels that can lead to insulin resistance. Moreover, diets rich in healthy fats, particularly omega-3 fatty acids found in fish, nuts, and seeds, can improve insulin sensitivity by reducing inflammation and supporting cell membrane health.

On the other hand, the modern penchant for processed foods, sugary beverages, and high-glycemic carbohydrates has created a landscape where blood sugar spikes are the norm rather than the exception. These dietary habits not only challenge the pancreas and its insulin-producing capacity but also disrupt the intricate balance of the body's metabolic processes. Thus, choosing whole, nutrient-dense foods over processed options is akin to choosing a path in the labyrinth that leads towards metabolic harmony and optimal health.

Intermittent fasting (IF) emerges as a powerful tool in this journey, offering a way to reset the body's sensitivity to insulin. By cycling between periods of eating and fasting, IF can help lower baseline insulin levels, improving the body's responsiveness to this critical hormone. This effect is akin to clearing the brush from a path, making it easier to navigate the metabolic maze. Moreover, the fasting periods encourage the body to shift from using glucose as its primary energy source to tapping into fat stores, further supporting blood sugar balance and metabolic health.

The synergy between diet, intermittent fasting, and lifestyle choices creates a foundation for balancing insulin and blood sugar levels. Physical activity, for instance, complements dietary efforts by enhancing insulin sensitivity and encouraging the muscles to use glucose more efficiently. Similarly, stress management and adequate sleep are critical components of this puzzle. Chronic stress and sleep deprivation can lead to elevated cortisol levels, which in turn can spike blood sugar levels and disrupt insulin sensitivity.

Embarking on the journey to balance insulin and blood sugar levels is a deeply personal endeavor, one that requires an understanding of one's body, lifestyle, and the unique challenges one faces. It's about more than just choosing the right foods or adopting intermittent fasting; it's about crafting a lifestyle that supports metabolic balance and overall health. This might mean prioritizing sleep, managing stress through mindfulness or meditation, engaging in regular physical activity, and, of course, making informed dietary choices that support insulin sensitivity.

In essence, balancing insulin and blood sugar levels is a journey of self-discovery and transformation. It's about navigating the complex interplay of diet, hormones, and lifestyle to find a path that leads to metabolic harmony and optimal health. This journey, while challenging, is replete with opportunities for growth, empowerment, and a deeper connection with the intricate workings of our bodies. It's a testament to the power of informed, intentional choices to shape our health and well-being, guiding us through the labyrinth of metabolic health towards a destination of vitality and balance.

Boosting Fat Burning Through Hormonal Optimization

Unlocking the full potential of our bodies to burn fat through hormonal optimization is not just a chapter in the vast book of wellness; it's a revolution in understanding how our bodies work and how we can work with them. This journey into boosting fat burning through hormonal optimization is akin to discovering a hidden pathway in our body's complex system, one that leads to enhanced health, vitality, and well-being. It's about fine-tuning our internal engines to burn fuel more efficiently, tapping into stored fat as a primary energy source, and doing so by leveraging the power of our hormones.

Our bodies are orchestrated by a symphony of hormones, each playing a specific role in regulating metabolism, appetite, and fat storage. Among these, insulin, cortisol, leptin, and thyroid hormones stand out as key conductors in the metabolic process. Insulin, as discussed, regulates blood sugar levels and affects fat storage. Cortisol, known as the stress hormone, can promote fat storage when levels are chronically high. Leptin signals satiety but can lead to leptin resistance in some cases, and thyroid hormones regulate metabolic rate. Balancing these hormones is crucial for optimizing fat burning.

Enhancing insulin sensitivity is foundational for boosting fat burning. When our cells are sensitive to insulin, glucose is efficiently transported from the bloodstream into cells, reducing the need for insulin and thereby lowering its levels.

Lower insulin levels allow the body to more easily access and burn stored fat. Dietary strategies to improve insulin sensitivity include reducing sugar intake, increasing fiber, and incorporating healthy fats and proteins into meals. These changes can help shift the body from a state of storing fat to one of burning it.

Cortisol plays a vital role in our body's response to stress. While it's essential for survival, chronic elevated cortisol levels can lead to increased appetite, cravings for sugar, and the accumulation of abdominal fat. Managing stress through mindfulness practices, adequate sleep, and regular physical activity can help normalize cortisol levels, thereby supporting the body's ability to burn fat more effectively.

Leptin resistance is a condition where the body does not respond properly to leptin signals, leading to increased hunger and a slower metabolism. Combating leptin resistance involves eating a nutrient-dense diet, avoiding inflammatory foods, and ensuring adequate sleep, as sleep deprivation can worsen leptin sensitivity. By restoring proper leptin function, we can help our body recognize satiety signals correctly and boost fat burning.

The thyroid gland produces hormones that regulate our metabolic rate. Ensuring optimal thyroid function is crucial for maintaining a metabolism that efficiently burns fat. Consuming adequate levels of iodine, found in seaweed and fish, selenium, found in Brazil nuts and sunflower seeds, and zinc, found in meat and lentils, can support thyroid health. Additionally, avoiding goitrogenic foods like raw cruciferous vegetables in excess can help maintain thyroid hormone production.

Intermittent fasting (IF) emerges as a potent strategy for hormonal optimization. IF can enhance insulin sensitivity, reduce leptin resistance, lower cortisol levels, and support healthy thyroid function. By cycling between periods of eating and fasting, IF helps the body recalibrate its hormonal responses, shifting the metabolism towards burning fat more efficiently.

Boosting fat burning through hormonal optimization requires a holistic approach that encompasses diet, lifestyle, and mindfulness practices. It's about creating a conducive environment for our hormones to function optimally, enabling our bodies to unlock the stored energy in fat cells and use it efficiently. This approach not only aids in weight management but also enhances overall health and well-being.

Optimizing our hormones for fat burning is a journey that transcends diet alone. It's a comprehensive approach that involves nurturing our bodies with the right foods, managing stress, ensuring restorative sleep, engaging in regular physical activity, and considering the timing of our meals through intermittent fasting. By understanding and respecting the intricate dance of hormones within our bodies, we can unlock our innate potential to burn fat more effectively, paving the way to improved health, energy, and vitality. This journey, while deeply personal, holds universal keys to unlocking a more vibrant, healthful life.

Dietary Strategies to Enhance Hormone Function

Crafting dietary strategies to enhance hormone function is akin to fine-tuning a high-performance engine, ensuring every component works in perfect harmony for optimal performance. In the realm of health and wellness, our hormones are the unsung heroes, orchestrating a myriad of bodily functions from metabolism to mood regulation. Understanding how to nourish our bodies to support this delicate hormonal balance is not just a chapter in our wellness journey; it's a fundamental pillar of a vibrant, healthful life.

At the heart of enhancing hormone function through diet lies the principle of balance. Just as a symphony requires the harmonious interplay of all its instruments, our bodies thrive on a balanced intake of macronutrients (proteins, fats, carbohydrates) and micronutrients (vitamins and minerals). Proteins provide the essential amino acids required for the production and function of many hormones. Healthy fats, particularly omega-3 fatty acids, play a crucial role in creating the cellular structure of hormones. Meanwhile, complex carbohydrates help regulate blood sugar levels, thereby influencing insulin sensitivity and overall hormonal balance.

Micronutrients wield immense power in the optimization of hormone function. Magnesium, for instance, is pivotal for the regulation of cortisol levels, helping to mitigate the effects of stress on the body. Zinc plays a critical role in the synthesis of hormones, including thyroid hormones and insulin. Vitamin D, often dubbed the "sunshine vitamin," is essential for the production of several hormones, including testosterone and estrogen. Ensuring a diet rich in these and other micronutrients supports the intricate web of hormonal activity that underpins our health.

Beyond macronutrients and micronutrients, phytonutrients—compounds found in fruits, vegetables, herbs, and spices—offer potent benefits for hormone function. For example, cruciferous vegetables such as broccoli and Brussels sprouts contain indole-3-carbinol, a compound that supports estrogen metabolism, aiding in the maintenance of hormonal equilibrium. Similarly, adaptogenic herbs like ashwagandha can modulate cortisol levels, enhancing the body's resilience to stress.

Intermittent fasting (IF) and other strategic eating patterns emerge as powerful tools in the dietary toolkit for hormone optimization. IF, by modulating the timing of food intake, can improve insulin sensitivity, reduce inflammation, and support the natural rhythms of hormone production, particularly growth hormone, which plays a key role in fat metabolism and muscle growth. Coupled with mindful eating practices, IF can help recalibrate the body's hormonal responses to food, fostering a more attuned and harmonious metabolic state.

The gut microbiome, with its vast population of beneficial bacteria, exerts a profound influence on hormone function. A diet rich in fiber, fermented foods, and prebiotics feeds the microbiome, promoting the production of short-chain fatty acids and other metabolites that can modulate hormonal activity. This gut-hormone axis is a testament to the interconnectedness of our dietary choices and our hormonal health, highlighting the importance of gut health in maintaining hormonal balance.

Enhancing hormone function through dietary strategies is a deeply personal endeavor, requiring an understanding of one's own body, lifestyle, and health goals. It involves not just the what of eating—choosing foods that support hormonal health—but also the how, embracing patterns of eating that align with our body's natural rhythms. This holistic approach, blending science with self-awareness, transforms our diet from mere sustenance to a powerful ally in our quest for health and vitality.

The journey to enhance hormone function through diet is a voyage of discovery, a process of learning how to nourish our bodies in a way that supports the complex, beautiful symphony of hormonal activity that animates our every moment. It's about making informed, mindful choices that elevate our well-being, enabling us to lead fuller, more vibrant lives. Through this lens, each meal becomes an opportunity to nurture not just our bodies, but our holistic health, weaving the art and science of nutrition into the fabric of our daily existence.

Part III: Mindset and Motivation

Cultivating a Positive Outlook

Setting Achievable Goals

The art of setting achievable goals lies in striking a balance between challenge and realism. It's a dance between dreaming big and anchoring those dreams in the tangible realities of our daily lives. This balance is crucial because goals that stretch us too thin can lead to frustration and burnout, while goals that don't challenge us enough might result in complacency and stagnation. The key is to find that sweet spot – goals that ignite our passion and drive without tipping us into overwhelm.

The first step in this delicate balancing act is a deep dive into self-reflection. Understanding our personal capacity involves an honest assessment of our current physical, mental, and emotional resources. It's about acknowledging our strengths and recognizing areas where we might need to grow or seek support. Similarly, aligning our goals with our desires means looking beyond the superficial to understand what truly motivates us. Is it the desire for health, longevity, connection, or perhaps the challenge itself? By anchoring our goals in our core values and desires, we ensure they resonate on a profound level, fueling our motivation over the long haul.

The SMART framework offers a practical approach to setting goals that are Specific, Measurable, Achievable, Relevant, and Time-bound. This method transforms vague aspirations into clear, actionable objectives. For instance, rather than setting a goal to "lose weight," a SMART goal would be to "lose 10 pounds in 90 days by incorporating intermittent fasting into my routine and exercising for at least 30 minutes three times a week." This level of specificity not only clarifies what success looks like but also outlines the path to achieve it, making the goal more tangible and within reach.

Achieving big goals often requires breaking them down into smaller, incremental steps. This strategy not only makes the goal more manageable but also provides opportunities for small victories along the way. These victories are crucial for maintaining motivation, as each one serves as a milestone, reminding us of our progress and reinforcing our commitment to the journey. For instance, if the goal is to adopt a 16/8 intermittent fasting regimen, starting with a 12-hour fasting window and gradually increasing it can help ease the transition, making the ultimate goal feel more attainable.

Life is unpredictable, and our initial plans may not always unfold as expected. Embracing flexibility in goal-setting means allowing room for adjustments along the way. This adaptability is not a sign of failure but a recognition of our dynamic nature and changing circumstances. It's about being kind to ourselves, understanding that progress is not always linear, and that sometimes, the path to our goals may need to be rerouted.

Setting achievable goals is intrinsically linked to cultivating a positive outlook. When our goals are aligned with our capacities, desires, and the realities of our lives, they become sources of inspiration rather than sources of stress. This positive outlook is self-reinforcing; as we meet our goals, our belief in our ability to effect change grows, further fueling our motivation and commitment to our journey of transformation.

In essence, setting achievable goals is the first step in a journey of self-discovery and growth. It's about laying a foundation for success that is rooted in self-awareness, strategic planning, and a positive mindset. As we navigate the challenges and triumphs of this journey, our goals serve as lighthouses, guiding us toward our best selves. They remind us that with each step forward, no matter how small, we are moving closer to realizing our vision for health, happiness, and fulfillment.

Building Resilience Against Setbacks

Embarking on a journey of self-improvement and personal growth requires an intricate dance between setting intentions, cultivating resilience, and fostering a supportive community, much like navigating a complex maze where each turn represents a choice or challenge that shapes our path forward. In this odyssey, the art of setting achievable goals emerges not just as a mere task but as a foundational pillar, akin to charting a course across uncharted waters with the stars as guides, illuminating aspirations that are both lofty and grounded in the reality of our daily lives. This delicate balance ensures that our goals stretch us, pushing the boundaries of what we believe possible while remaining firmly rooted in the achievable, thus avoiding the pitfalls of frustration and burnout. The essence of building resilience against setbacks lies in transforming our perspective, viewing obstacles not as insurmountable walls but as stepping stones on the path to growth and learning. It's about embracing a growth mindset, which thrives on challenge and views failure not as a mark of defeat but as a springboard for development and a testament to our evolving capabilities. Cultivating resilience involves a multi-faceted approach, integrating reflection, realistic expectations, self-compassion, flexible problem-solving, and emotional regulation into our toolkit, each strategy weaving into the fabric of our resilience like threads in a tapestry. Central to this journey is the support of a community, a collective that not only provides a sounding board for our challenges but also serves as a mirror reflecting our progress, offering encouragement, perspective, and wisdom gleaned from shared experiences. This interplay between personal endeavor and communal support underscores the notion that while our journey of self-improvement is deeply personal, it is also inextricably linked to the fabric of our relationships and the communities we inhabit. As we navigate this journey, we learn that setbacks are not detours but integral parts of our narrative, each one offering lessons that enrich our understanding and fortify our resolve. This holistic approach to personal growth, blending the setting of achievable goals, the cultivation of resilience, and the nurturing of supportive relationships, transcends the sum of its parts, evolving into a transformative process that propels us toward our most authentic selves, equipped with the wisdom, strength, and support to navigate the complexities of life with grace, purpose, and an unwavering commitment to continual growth and self-discovery. This continuum of growth and self-discovery, then, is not a linear path but a spiral, ever-expanding and deepening, where each cycle of setting goals, encountering setbacks, and leaning on our community teaches us more about our resilience, our capacities, and the interconnectedness of our journeys. As we delve deeper into this process, we uncover layers of our potential that were previously obscured, revealing not just our ability to achieve what we set out to do but also our capacity for adaptation, for empathy, and for profound transformation. This realization that our goals, challenges, and support systems are not just checkpoints or lifelines but integral parts of a larger tapestry of human experience enriches our journey, adding a depth of meaning and purpose that transcends the individual achievements or setbacks. It's in this rich soil of understanding and connection that true growth occurs, where the seeds of our aspirations take root, strengthened by the nourishment of our resilience and the sunlight of our community's support, blossoming into expressions of our deepest selves. Through this ongoing cycle of striving, learning, and connecting, we not only move closer to our individual ideals of success and fulfillment but also contribute to the collective growth of our communities, inspiring and uplifting those around us with the stories of our challenges, our resilience, and our unwavering pursuit of a life lived fully and authentically. Thus, the journey of self-improvement and personal growth unfolds as an endless horizon, where each step forward, each setback navigated, and each hand held in support is a testament to the beauty and complexity of human potential, a reminder that our capacity for growth is boundless, and that the journey itself, with all its twists and turns, is where the true magic of transformation lies.

The Importance of Community and Support

In the grand tapestry of personal growth and self-improvement, the threads of community and support are not just complementary; they are essential. This realization brings to light the profound impact of our social connections on our journey towards cultivating a positive outlook. The significance of community and support in our lives cannot be overstated—it's akin to finding a harbor in a storm, offering shelter, guidance, and the strength to sail forth once more.

The essence of community lies in its ability to reflect back to us not just who we are, but who we aspire to be. It's in the shared stories, the collective struggles, and the communal triumphs that we find the courage to set goals and the resilience to navigate setbacks. Community acts as a mirror, reflecting our potential for growth and the possibility of transformation that lies within each of us. This reflection is not merely about validation but about inspiration—a call to action that resonates with the core of our being, urging us to move beyond our perceived limitations.

Support, in its many forms, is the cornerstone upon which the edifice of personal development is built. It's the encouraging word from a friend that reignites our motivation, the wisdom of a mentor that guides our path, or the empathetic ear of a confidant that helps us navigate the complexities of our emotions. Support is multifaceted—it's both the tangible assistance that helps us overcome immediate obstacles and the intangible sense of belonging that nurtures our inner strength. The synergy between community and support fosters a nurturing environment in which individuals can flourish. This environment acts as a greenhouse for personal growth, where the seeds of potential are watered with encouragement and the sunlight of collective wisdom promotes growth. In this space, the journey of setting achievable goals and building resilience against setbacks is shared, not solitary. It's a collaborative endeavor where success is celebrated as a collective achievement, and setbacks are met with a chorus of support, reminding us that we are not alone.

Moreover, the role of community and support in cultivating a positive outlook extends beyond the individual. It creates a ripple effect, where the growth and transformation of one person inspire and catalyze change in others. This ripple effect underscores the interconnectedness of our journeys, highlighting how our individual actions contribute to a larger narrative of communal growth and positive change.

In navigating the challenges of life, the importance of community and support reminds us that our strength often comes from the connections we forge with others. These connections provide a foundation of stability and a source of limitless potential. They remind us that every setback is an opportunity for growth, not just for the individual but for the community as a whole. They teach us that our goals, no matter how personal, are part of a collective aspiration towards a more fulfilled, resilient, and connected existence.

In essence, the journey towards cultivating a positive outlook, underpinned by the setting of achievable goals and the building of resilience, is profoundly enriched by the embrace of community and support. This journey, marked by the milestones of personal achievement and the waypoints of collective encouragement, is a testament to the human spirit's capacity for growth, transformation, and profound connection. It reaffirms the belief that together, we can navigate the complexities of life, turning challenges into opportunities for growth and setbacks into stepping stones for progress. In this shared journey, the importance of community and support shines as a beacon of hope, guiding us towards a future where personal fulfillment and collective well-being are inextricably linked, empowering us to become not just the best versions of ourselves but also steadfast allies in the growth of those around us.

Mental Clarity and Emotional Well-being

The Psychological Benefits of Intermittent Dieting

Intermittent fasting reveals a landscape rich with psychological benefits, where the terrain is as varied and profound as the human mind itself. This path, less traveled by those seeking mental clarity and emotional well-being, offers more than just a method for managing weight; it's a gateway to a deeper understanding of our relationship with food, our bodies, and our minds. At the heart of intermittent fasting lies the practice of cycling between periods of eating and not eating, a rhythm that echoes the natural ebb and flow of life itself. This rhythm, when embraced, can lead to a remarkable shift in how we experience hunger, satisfaction, and ultimately, how we interact with the world around us. The psychological benefits of this practice are manifold, beginning with an enhanced sense of control over one's eating habits. This control is not about restriction but about empowerment, a reclaiming of agency over when and how we nourish our bodies. It's a profound shift from eating out of habit or emotion to eating with intention, a change that can lead to a more mindful relationship with food. This mindfulness, in turn, fosters a heightened awareness of our bodies' hunger and satiety signals, leading us to a place where we can distinguish between physical hunger and emotional hunger, between eating to live and living to eat. The journey through intermittent fasting also leads to increased mental clarity, as periods of not eating can reduce the mental fog and lethargy often associated with constant eating or overeating. This clarity is not merely about the absence of food but about the presence of space—space for our bodies to rest and repair, and space for our minds to breathe and expand. In this space, we often find a wellspring of creativity, focus, and productivity, as if fasting clears not just the physical clutter but the mental clutter as well. Moreover, the discipline and structure inherent in intermittent fasting can spill over into other areas of life, fostering a sense of accomplishment and resilience that extends beyond the dining table. This practice teaches us that we are capable of enduring discomfort, of waiting, of delaying gratification for greater rewards. It's a lesson in patience and persistence, virtues that are as valuable in achieving our goals as they are in navigating the challenges of life. Yet, perhaps one of the most profound psychological benefits of intermittent fasting is the journey inward it necessitates. This journey is one of self-discovery, of confronting our habits, our cravings, and our fears. It's a journey that asks us to sit with discomfort, to listen to our bodies, and to question the stories we've been told about food, hunger, and satisfaction. This self-reflection can lead to a deeper understanding of our emotional eating patterns, our triggers, and our coping mechanisms, offering a pathway not just to better physical health but to emotional and psychological healing. In essence, the psychological benefits of intermittent fasting are a tapestry woven from threads of mindfulness, self-control, mental clarity, discipline, resilience, and self-discovery. It's a practice that challenges us to rethink our relationship with food and with ourselves, offering a mirror in which we can see not just our physical reflection but our mental and emotional landscapes. As we walk this path, we find that intermittent fasting is not just a diet or a health trend but a journey of transformation, a journey that has the power to change not just how we eat, but how we live, think, and feel.

Managing Stress Without Food

In our modern landscape, stress has become a constant companion for many. Often, we turn to food as a source of comfort, a momentary escape from the pressures and anxieties that weigh us down. However, this strategy can be counterproductive, leading to a cycle of stress eating that only temporarily masks the underlying issues. Learning to manage stress without using food as a crutch is a vital skill, one that empowers us to navigate life's challenges with resilience and grace.

The first step in this journey is recognizing the patterns that link stress to our eating habits. It requires a mindful awareness of the moments when we reach for food not out of hunger but as an emotional response to stress. This awareness is the foundation upon which we can build new, healthier coping mechanisms.

One effective strategy is engaging in regular physical activity. Exercise is a powerful stress reliever, known to reduce levels of the body's stress hormones, such as adrenaline and cortisol, while simultaneously stimulating the production of endorphins, the body's natural mood elevators. Whether it's a brisk walk, a yoga session, or a vigorous workout, physical activity provides a healthy outlet for stress, redirecting the energy that might otherwise lead us to seek comfort in food.

Another key approach is practicing mindfulness and meditation. These practices help us cultivate a state of present-moment awareness, allowing us to observe our thoughts and feelings without judgment. By becoming more attuned to our inner experiences, we can better recognize the onset of stress and choose responses that serve our well-being, rather than defaulting to food for emotional relief.

Deepening our social connections offers another path to managing stress. Sharing our concerns, joys, and struggles with friends, family, or support groups can provide a sense of relief and belonging. Social support acts as a buffer against stress, reminding us that we're not alone in our experiences. It's in these connections that we often find comfort and perspective, alleviating the need to seek solace in eating.

Cultivating hobbies and interests outside of our daily routines can also serve as a valuable stress management tool. Engaging in activities that bring us joy and fulfillment—be it painting, gardening, playing music, or any other pursuit—can provide a much-needed distraction from stressors, enriching our lives and reducing the temptation to turn to food for comfort.

Lastly, ensuring adequate rest and sleep is crucial in the fight against stress. Sleep deprivation can exacerbate stress and negatively impact our emotional resilience. By prioritizing sleep, we equip our bodies and minds to handle stress more effectively, reducing the likelihood of stress-induced eating.

Managing stress without food is about building a toolkit of strategies that address the root causes of stress, rather than masking them with temporary comforts. It's a holistic approach that encompasses physical activity, mindfulness, social connection, engaging in passions, and prioritizing rest. Through these practices, we can navigate the complexities of life with a clearer mind and a more balanced emotional state, freeing ourselves from the cycle of stress eating and moving towards a place of greater health, happiness, and well-being.

In the intricate dance of life where stress undeniably takes center stage for many, the act of reaching for food as a source of comfort has become a well-rehearsed routine. This routine, though momentarily soothing, often leads to a counterproductive cycle of stress eating, serving only to maskthe deeper issues at hand rather than addressing them. To break free from this cycle, it's imperative to develop strategies for managing stress that don't involve using food as a crutch. This endeavor not only fosters mental clarity and emotional well-being but also empowers us to face life's challenges with a resilience that is both graceful and robust.

The journey towards mastering stress without the aid of comfort food begins with the critical step of pattern recognition. It demands a mindful awareness and an honest acknowledgment of the instances when food is sought not out of genuine hunger but as an emotional balm for stress. This realization lays the groundwork for the cultivation of healthier coping mechanisms, strategies that address the root of stress without the temporary fix food provides.

Engaging in regular physical activity emerges as a potent antidote to stress. The benefits of exercise extend far beyond the physical, acting as a powerful catalyst for the reduction of the body's stress hormones, such as adrenaline and cortisol, and the amplification of endorphins, those natural mood-enhancing chemicals that promote a sense of well-being. The beauty of physical activity as a stress management tool lies in its versatility—whether it's the rhythmic calm of a yoga session, the endorphin rush of a high-intensity workout, or the simple joy of a brisk walk in nature, each form of exercise offers a unique pathway to stress relief.

Mindfulness and meditation offer another avenue for

managing stress, one that emphasizes the power of present-moment awareness. These practices invite us to engage deeply with our current experience, observing thoughts and emotions without judgment. This heightened state of awareness enables us to identify the onset of stress and consciously choose how to respond, shifting our default from seeking solace in food to finding peace within the moment.

The role of social connections in managing stress cannot be overstated. In sharing our lives—our triumphs and trials—with friends, family, or support groups, we find a sense of relief and belonging that food simply cannot replicate. These connections serve as a lifeline, a reminder that we are not isolated in our experiences but part of a larger, supportive community. It's within the safety of these relationships that we can find true comfort and perspective, diminishing the lure of emotional eating.

Moreover, the pursuit of hobbies and interests offers a fulfilling escape from the stresses of daily life. Immersing ourselves in activities that bring joy and satisfaction provides a distraction from stressors and enriches our lives in meaningful ways, reducing the impulse to turn to food for comfort.

The significance of adequate rest and sleep in the battle against stress deserves emphasis. Sleep deprivation not only magnifies stress but also impairs our emotional resilience, making stress-induced eating more likely. By prioritizing sleep, we arm ourselves with the strength to face stress head

-on, equipped with a clearer mind and a more balanced emotional state.

In conclusion, managing stress without resorting to food involves a holistic strategy that embraces physical activity, mindfulness, meaningful social interactions, the pursuit of personal passions, and the prioritization of rest. This comprehensive approach addresses the underlying causes of stress, enabling us to navigate life's complexities with enhanced mental clarity and emotional equilibrium. Through these practices, we can liberate ourselves from the cycle of stress eating and step into a realm of greater health, happiness, and overall well-being, marking a profound shift in how we cope with stress and enriching our lives in ways we never thought possible.

Enhancing Mood Through Nutrition

The intricate relationship between what we eat and how we feel is both fascinating and profound. Nutrition plays a pivotal role not just in our physical health but in our mental and emotional states as well. This connection, deeply rooted in the biochemistry of our brains and bodies, offers a powerful avenue for enhancing mood and overall well-being through dietary choices. By understanding and leveraging this connection, we can significantly impact our daily experiences of happiness, energy, and emotional resilience.

At the heart of this relationship are the nutrients that act as the building blocks for neurotransmitters, the brain's chemical messengers responsible for our emotions, thoughts, and feelings. For instance, omega-3 fatty acids, found in fatty fish, flaxseeds, and walnuts, are crucial for brain health, playing a role in enhancing mood and combating depression. These essential fats contribute to the fluidity of brain cell membranes, facilitating the efficient transmission of neurotransmitter signals.

Similarly, amino acids, the components of proteins, serve as precursors to neurotransmitters involved in mood regulation. Tryptophan, for example, is a precursor to serotonin, often dubbed the "feel-good" neurotransmitter. Foods rich in tryptophan, such as turkey, eggs, and cheese, can thus support serotonin production and positively influence mood.

Complex carbohydrates are another dietary component with a significant impact on mood. By promoting a steady release of glucose into the bloodstream, complex carbs ensure a consistent energy supply to the brain, preventing the mood dips associated with blood sugar spikes and crashes. Furthermore, these carbohydrates can increase the level of serotonin in the brain, providing a natural mood boost.

The role of vitamins and minerals in mood regulation is also critical. Vitamins B6 and B12, folate, and magnesium, for instance, play key roles in the synthesis and function of neurotransmitters. Deficiencies in these nutrients have been linked to increased risk of depression and mood disorders. A diet rich in leafy greens, legumes, nuts, and whole grains can help ensure adequate intake of these essential nutrients.

Hydration is another often overlooked aspect of nutrition that can significantly affect mood and cognitive function. Even mild dehydration can impair concentration, increase irritability, and lead to a decline in mood. Ensuring adequate fluid intake is a simple yet effective strategy for maintaining optimal mental and emotional well-being.

In addition to what we eat, how we eat also matters. Regular, balanced meals and snacks can help maintain stable blood sugar levels, providing a consistent energy source for the brain and preventing mood swings. Mindful eating practices, where attention is given to the experience of eating, can enhance the enjoyment and satisfaction derived from food, further contributing to a positive mood.

In essence, enhancing mood through nutrition is about more than just eating the right foods; it's about embracing a holistic approach to diet that recognizes the profound impact of nutrition on our mental and emotional landscapes. By making informed, mindful dietary choices, we can support our brain's biochemistry in a way that promotes mental clarity, emotional balance, and an overall sense of well-being. This journey towards a mood-enhancing diet is a testament to the power of nutrition as a tool for nurturing not just the body but the mind and spirit as well.

Part IV: Integrating Movement

Exercise for Empowerment

Tailoring Physical Activity to Your Body's Needs

As we begin the process of incorporating movement into our lives—especially for women over 50—we are getting closer to the point where physical activity ceases to be merely a routine and instead becomes a transformational force. This is the time in life to reconnect with our bodies, to pay attention and act appropriately. This is the core of adjusting your exercise regimen to your body's demands; this is a process that calls for focus, compassion, and a thorough comprehension of the particular rhythms and changes our bodies go through at this point in life. For women stepping into the empowerment of their later years, the narrative around exercise shifts from the pursuit of high-intensity, calorie-torching workouts to fostering a harmonious balance that honors the body's current state and future well-being. It's about crafting a regimen that aligns with your life's rhythms, one that feels like a natural extension of your day rather than an imposition.

The concept of tailoring physical activity is deeply rooted in the principle of self-awareness. It begins with a conversation, a series of gentle inquiries we pose to ourselves. What movements bring joy and invigoration? How does my body feel today, and what does it need to thrive? This dialogue is the foundation upon which a personalized fitness journey is built, recognizing that the answer may evolve from one day to the next.

Understanding the physiological nuances of aging is paramount. Our bodies, after crossing the threshold of 50, are in a state of graceful transformation. The metabolism adjusts, muscle mass naturally declines, and joints might whisper tales of discomfort if not cared for properly. Yet, this is not a narrative of decline but an invitation to adapt and flourish. Tailoring physical activity means embracing low-impact exercises that protect the joints while effectively enhancing cardiovascular health, like swimming or cycling. It's about discovering the potency of resistance training, which counteracts muscle loss and fortifies bones, without the necessity for heavy lifting that might stress the body.

Moreover, the integration of movement into daily life becomes an art form. It's the subtle choices that weave a tapestry of wellness: opting for stairs over elevators, engaging in gardening or dance, and transforming mundane tasks into opportunities for gentle stretching and strength building. This philosophy extends beyond structured exercise; it's a holistic approach that cherishes movement in all its forms, acknowledging that every step, every bend, contributes to our vitality.

Flexibility and balance, both physical and metaphorical, are pillars of this tailored approach. Incorporating practices like yoga or Tai Chi not only enhances physical flexibility but also instills a sense of mental calm and balance, offering a sanctuary from the whirlwind of daily life. These practices underscore the importance of breath, of moving with intention and grace, fostering a connection between mind, body, and spirit that is especially nurturing for women navigating the nuances of menopause and beyond.

The journey of tailoring physical activity is also one of experimentation and curiosity. It invites exploration—perhaps rediscovering a long-forgotten sport or hobby, or the thrill of trying something entirely new. This exploration is guided by the wisdom of our bodies, which communicate their preferences and limits in subtle yet unmistakable signals. It's a path marked by patience and kindness towards oneself, acknowledging that progress is not measured by the sweat on our brow but by the joy in our hearts and the strength in our bodies.

Empowerment through exercise, at its core, is about crafting a narrative of self-care that defies the conventional scripts of aging. It's a commitment to living fully, to embracing the present with vigor and looking to the future with anticipation. This approach fosters resilience, enabling us to meet life's challenges with grace and agility, to dance through the rain, and to stand strong against the gusts of change.

Tailoring physical activity to your body's needs is, ultimately, a celebration of life. It's an affirmation that age is not a barrier but a horizon, rich with potential and beauty. It is an act of self-love and a testament to the enduring strength of the female spirit. As we embark on this path, we do so with the knowledge that our journey is as unique as we are, guided by the rhythms of our own bodies and the desires of our hearts. In this tailored approach to movement, we find not just health and vitality but a deeper connection to the essence of who we are, embracing each day with courage, joy, and an unwavering commitment to our well-being.

Strength Training: The Foundation of Youth

In the tapestry of aging gracefully, strength training emerges as the golden thread, weaving resilience and vitality into the fabric of our lives. For women over 50, it stands as a bastion against the tide of time, a foundation of youth that bolsters not just the body, but the spirit and mind as well. Embracing strength training is not merely about building muscle; it's a profound declaration of taking control, of asserting agency over our physical and emotional well-being.

At the heart of strength training lies a transformative power, one that transcends the conventional boundaries of exercise.

It's a journey that begins with the acknowledgment of our body's evolving needs, recognizing that the strength we build is not for vanity, but for life. This form of exercise becomes a beacon of empowerment, illuminating a path to a stronger, more resilient self. It challenges the narrative of decline that often shadows the years beyond 50, replacing it with a story of growth, strength, and enduring vitality.

Strength training, in its essence, is about connection. It's about forging a deeper relationship with our bodies, learning to communicate through movement, to listen to the whispers and roars of our muscles and joints. This dialogue is not always easy. It requires patience, understanding, and a willingness to adapt. But the rewards are immeasurable, offering not just physical gains but a profound sense of achievement and self-respect.

For women venturing into or living in the golden years of post-50, strength training holds a promise of independence. It fortifies the body against the vulnerabilities of age, such as osteoporosis and muscle atrophy, enabling us to move through our days with confidence and grace. But beyond the physical, it strengthens the sinews of our self-esteem, weaving resilience into our very identity. Each lift, each press, becomes a testament to our strength, not just as individuals, but as part of a community of women who refuse to be defined by age.

The approach to strength training at this stage of life is nuanced. It's not about the heaviest weights or the most repetitions, but about finding balance and harmony within our capabilities. It's a practice that values consistency over intensity, recognizing that the goal is not to compete, but to nurture and sustain. This perspective shifts the focus from external metrics of success to internal measures of wellness and satisfaction.

Incorporating strength training into our lives is also an act of creativity. It invites us to explore various modalities, from free weights and resistance bands to bodyweight exercises and machines. This exploration is guided by curiosity and a spirit of experimentation, finding joy in the process of discovery. It's a reminder that our fitness journey is deeply personal, a unique narrative that we author with each movement.

Moreover, strength training is a celebration of capability. It challenges the stereotypes and societal expectations that seek to confine women, particularly as they age. By engaging in this practice, we not only reclaim our physical agency but also challenge the cultural narratives around aging. We become embodiments of strength and resilience, inspiring not just our peers but younger generations to view aging through a lens of possibility and power.

The benefits of strength training extend into the fabric of our daily lives. It enhances our functional fitness, enabling us to lift groceries, play with grandchildren, and navigate the physical demands of our routines with ease and agility. But perhaps more significantly, it cultivates a mindset of empowerment. It teaches us that we are capable of change, that our actions have power, and that age is but a number, not a limit.

As we integrate strength training into our lives, we embark on a journey of transformation. It's a path that challenges us, that asks us to embrace discomfort in the pursuit of growth. But it's also a journey of joy, of celebrating our strength and marveling at our body's capacity to adapt and thrive. In this practice, we find not just a foundation of youth but a source of enduring empowerment, a testament to our resilience, and a celebration of our unwavering spirit.

Strength training for women over 50 is not just about physical fitness; it's a powerful avenue for self-discovery and empowerment. It's about rewriting the narrative of aging, proving that every year brings with it an opportunity for growth and renewal. As we lift, press, and grow stronger, we do so with the knowledge that we are building more than muscle; we are forging a legacy of strength, vitality, and indomitable spirit.

Gentle Mobility: Yoga and Pilates for Flexibility

In the golden years of life, the journey towards empowerment through exercise takes a gentle, yet profoundly impactful turn towards the realms of yoga and Pilates. These practices, rooted in the principles of mindfulness, flexibility, and core strength, offer a sanctuary for women over 50 to explore movement in a way that nurtures both the body and soul. They stand as pillars of gentle mobility, guiding us towards a harmony of physical and mental well-being, a place where flexibility transcends the physical, weaving into the very fabric of our resilience and adaptability in life.

Yoga and Pilates are more than mere exercises; they are dialogues between the body and breath, a dance of grace and strength that resonates deeply with the rhythms of our mature selves. They beckon us to slow down, to listen intently to the whispers of our bodies, and to honor our journey with each stretch, each pose, and each breath. This practice of gentle mobility is a celebration of what our bodies can do, of the space we occupy in the world, and of the fluidity with which we can move through the various stages of life.

The essence of integrating yoga and Pilates into our lives as we age is not about achieving the perfect pose or mastering complex sequences. It's about the journey towards inner strength, about finding balance and grounding in a world that often feels in constant flux. These practices teach us to embrace our vulnerabilities, to see them as opportunities for growth and self-discovery. They remind us that flexibility is not just a physical attribute but a mindset, a way of being that embraces change with grace and courage.

For women over 50, yoga and Pilates serve as a gateway to empowerment through the cultivation of a deep, intrinsic strength that supports the spine of our existence. They offer a pathway to reclaiming our bodies, to stepping into our power with confidence and poise. Through the practice of gentle mobility, we learn to move with intention, to breathe through challenges, and to stand tall amidst the storms of life. These practices become a metaphor for our resilience, a testament to our ability to bend without breaking, to flow with the currents of life with elegance and strength.

Yoga, with its rich tapestry of styles and philosophies, offers a myriad of paths to explore. From the gentle flows of Hatha yoga, which soothe and strengthen the body with a focus on alignment and breath, to the restorative poses of Yin yoga, which delve deep into the connective tissues, inviting a release of long-held tensions. Each style of yoga provides a unique lens through which to view and engage with our bodies and minds, offering insights and experiences that are as varied and rich as life itself.

Pilates, on the other hand, brings a focused attention to the core, the powerhouse of the body, from which all movement emanates. It teaches precision, control, and the art of moving with efficiency and grace. Pilates is not just about physical strength; it's about cultivating a balanced body, a sharp mind, and a spirit attuned to the subtleties of movement and breath. It's a practice that builds not just muscle, but confidence and a deep, resonant joy in the capabilities of our bodies.

Integrating yoga and Pilates into our lives is an act of self-care, a declaration of worthiness, and a commitment to nurturing ourselves in a holistic and profound way. It's about carving out space and time to connect with ourselves, to honor our needs and our journey. This practice of gentle mobility becomes a source of strength and empowerment, a foundation upon which we can build a vibrant, fulfilling life.

As we navigate the complexities of aging, yoga and Pilates stand as steadfast companions, guiding us towards a deeper understanding of our bodies and our capacity for resilience, adaptability, and joy. They teach us to approach life with a sense of curiosity, to embrace the beauty of the present moment, and to move through the world with a sense of grace and empowerment.

The practice of gentle mobility through yoga and Pilates is not just about maintaining flexibility or enhancing physical health; it's about cultivating a life of balance, harmony, and profound well-being. It's about embracing the journey of aging with courage and grace, about living our lives with a sense of purpose, passion, and deep connection to the essence of who we are. Through these practices, we find not only a path to physical vitality but a gateway to a richer, more empowered life.

Staying Active in Everyday Life

Incorporating Movement into Your Routine

In the tapestry of our daily lives, movement weaves through each moment, an undercurrent that shapes our well-being, our vitality, and our connection to the world around us. For women over 50, incorporating movement into the routine is not just about physical health; it's a profound engagement with life itself, a declaration of presence and participation in every breath, every step. This chapter delves into the art of seamlessly blending movement into our daily lives, transforming the mundane into a dance of joy and empowerment.

At the heart of integrating movement into our daily routine is the recognition of its intrinsic value, not just as a means to an end but as a celebration of capability and resilience. Movement becomes a language through which we communicate with our bodies, a dialogue that honors our strengths and acknowledges our limitations with grace and compassion. It's about finding the rhythm in our daily tasks, the dance in our steps, and the joy in every movement, big or small.

The journey of weaving movement into the fabric of our daily lives begins with a shift in perspective. It's about seeing the potential for activity in the ordinary, the opportunities for engagement in the seemingly mundane. This shift invites us to explore the spaces between our obligations, to find moments of movement that not only enhance our physical health but enrich our lives with a sense of purpose and delight.

Incorporating movement into our routine is as much about creativity as it is about intention. It's about reimagining our daily tasks as opportunities for engagement and interaction with our environment. From the way we approach household chores to how we navigate our workspaces, every aspect of our day offers a canvas for integrating movement. It's transforming gardening into a practice of mindful movement, seeing the stretch and bend of tending to the earth as a dance of connection with nature. It's in the deliberate choice to take the stairs, to park a little further from the store entrance, to stand and stretch during long periods of sitting. Each choice is a step towards a more vibrant, engaged life.

Moreover, integrating movement into our daily lives is about breaking down the barriers between "exercise" and "living." It's recognizing that movement doesn't have to be compartmentalized into designated hours at the gym or morning runs. Instead, it's a thread that runs through the entirety of our day, enriching every moment with potential for strength, flexibility, and endurance. This holistic approach demystifies exercise, making it more accessible and woven into the very essence of our daily existence.

This practice of daily movement is also an exercise in mindfulness. It's about being present in our bodies, aware of our movements, and attuned to the messages our physical selves send us. This awareness builds a foundation of self-care and respect, guiding us towards activities that nourish and sustain us. It invites us to engage with movement not as a task but as a form of self-expression, a way to celebrate our journey, our challenges, and our triumphs.

Incorporating movement into our daily routine also fosters a sense of community and connection. It encourages us to seek out shared activities, to walk with friends, to join group classes not just for the exercise but for the joy of shared experience, of laughter and support and mutual growth. It's in these moments of connection that movement transcends the physical, becoming a catalyst for building relationships and fostering a sense of belonging.

As we navigate the path of integrating movement into our lives, we encounter the inevitable challenges and obstacles. Yet, it's in the facing of these challenges that we discover our resilience, our capacity for adaptation and change. We learn to modify activities to fit our needs, to listen to our bodies and respect their limits, and to find joy in the adaptations that make movement possible and enjoyable at any stage of life.

Incorporating movement into our daily routine is, ultimately, an act of empowerment. It's a declaration that we are active participants in our health and well-being, that we choose to engage with life fully, with vigor, and with joy. It's a practice that reminds us of our strength, our flexibility, and our endless capacity for growth. As we weave movement into the fabric of our daily lives, we do so with the knowledge that each step, each stretch, each moment of activity is a step towards a richer, more vibrant life.

In this dance of daily movement, we find not just health and vitality but a profound connection to the essence of who we are. We discover that movement is not just about physical fitness but about living fully, embracing each moment with a spirit of joy and a heart full of courage. It's in this integration of movement into our daily lives that we find the true essence of empowerment, a path that leads us not just towards better health but towards a deeper engagement with the world around us.

Fun and Engaging Activities for Every Fitness Level

In a world that often celebrates the fast-paced and the extreme, finding fun and engaging activities that cater to every fitness level can seem like a quest for the Holy Grail. Yet, the beauty of movement lies in its diversity, its ability to be molded and adapted to fit the unique journey of each individual. For women over 50, this quest becomes an exploration of joy, a rediscovery of play, and an embrace of activities that not only challenge the body but also invigorate the spirit and engage the mind.

At the core of this exploration is the understanding that movement should bring joy. It should be a source of pleasure, not a chore or a box to be checked off in the daily routine. This perspective shifts the approach to exercise from a task to a treat, transforming the way we view physical activity. It's about finding activities that light up our hearts, that make us smile as we move, and that leave us feeling refreshed and energized, not just physically, but emotionally and mentally as well.

Fun and engaging activities come in an array of colors and flavors, each offering its own unique benefits and joys. For some, this might mean dancing to the rhythm of their favorite tunes in the living room, feeling the music flow through them as they let go of inhibitions and simply move. For others, it could be the gentle, rhythmic stroke of a paddle as they kayak across a serene lake, the water whispering tales of tranquility and strength with each stroke.

Walking groups provide not only a way to stay active but also a means to connect with others, sharing stories and laughter as the miles pass underfoot. These groups offer a sense of community and support, a shared journey towards health that is enriched by the bonds of friendship and the beauty of the natural world. Whether it's a brisk walk through the neighborhood, a hike through the trails of a local park, or a leisurely stroll along the beach, walking becomes an adventure, a treasure hunt for beauty in the ordinary.

Cycling offers another avenue for exploration and enjoyment. The feeling of freedom as the wind caresses your face, the sense of accomplishment as you conquer a challenging hill, and the joy of exploring new paths and sceneries. Cycling can be adapted to various fitness levels, from leisurely rides on flat, scenic routes to more challenging terrains that test endurance and strength.

For those who seek the thrill of competition in a friendly, supportive environment, community sports leagues offer a chance to engage in team sports like volleyball, tennis, or pickleball. These activities not only provide a great workout but also foster a sense of camaraderie and competition, pushing you to reach new heights of fitness and skill in a fun, engaging way.

Gardening, too, is a celebration of movement, a dance of life that engages the body in bending, lifting, and stretching as you nurture the earth. It offers a unique blend of physical activity, creativity, and the joy of watching something grow – a testament to the beauty of life and the power of care and dedication.

Yoga and Pilates classes tailored to different levels of experience and flexibility offer a space to explore the limits of your body, to stretch and strengthen muscles you never knew you had, and to find balance and peace in the flow of movement and breath.

Exploring new forms of exercise, such as aqua aerobics, Zumba, or tai chi, can also add a refreshing variety to your routine, offering the excitement of learning and the joy of discovering movements that feel good to your body and soul.

Incorporating fun and engaging activities into your life is about writing your own story of movement, one that is filled with joy, exploration, and the celebration of what your body can do. It's about moving away from the shoulds and musts of exercise and stepping into a space of want and delight. This approach transforms the journey of staying active into an adventure, a daily dose of play and pleasure that enriches your life in ways far beyond the physical.

At the heart of this journey is the message that movement is a gift, an expression of gratitude to our bodies for the incredible work they do. It's an acknowledgment that staying active is not just about prolonging life but about enriching it, about filling each day with moments of joy, connection, and discovery. In this exploration of fun and engaging activities, we find not just health and vitality but a deeper engagement with the world around us, a celebration of life in all its vibrant, beautiful complexity.

Part V: Nutrition and Cooking for Vitality

Eating for Energy

Nutrient-Dense Foods for Women Over 50

In the vibrant tapestry of life after 50, nutrition plays a pivotal role in painting a picture of health that is as rich and varied as the experiences that women in this age group cherish. Eating for energy, especially for women over 50, transcends the mere act of satisfying hunger. It becomes a deliberate choice, a way to infuse each day with vitality, to fuel the body with the zest needed to embrace life's adventures. This journey into the world of nutrient-dense foods is not just about selecting the right ingredients; it's about weaving a kaleidoscope of flavors, textures, and nutrients that together form the foundation of a vibrant, energetic life.

Nutrient-dense foods are the superheroes of the dietary world for women over 50. They pack a powerful punch of vitamins, minerals, fiber, and antioxidants into each bite, without an excess of calories. These foods are the building blocks of a diet that supports energy levels, fortifies the body against age-related changes, and nourishes the soul with every delicious, carefully chosen morsel.

The cornerstone of this nutritional philosophy is variety. Just as a painter uses a spectrum of colors to bring a canvas to life, a well-rounded diet includes a rainbow of fruits and vegetables, each color representing a different suite of nutrients. Dark leafy greens, vibrant berries, deep purple eggplants, and bright orange carrots each contribute their unique blend of phytonutrients, fiber, and vitamins, painting a picture of health that is as pleasing to the eye as it is to the body.

Protein, too, plays a starring role in the diet of a woman over 50. As the body ages, maintaining muscle mass becomes crucial for sustaining energy, supporting metabolism, and ensuring mobility. Lean proteins such as fish, poultry, legumes, and plant-based alternatives provide the essential amino acids needed to rebuild and repair muscle tissue, fueling the body's energy engines and supporting an active, vibrant lifestyle.

Healthy fats are another key player in the nutrient-dense diet. Far from the villains they were once thought to be, fats like those found in avocados, nuts, seeds, and olive oil are vital for absorbing vitamins, supporting brain health, and keeping hunger at bay. These fats provide a slow, steady source of energy, keeping you fueled for the adventures that await.

Whole grains and seeds offer a bounty of nutrition, including B vitamins, which are essential for converting food into energy.

Quinoa, barley, oats, and chia seeds are just a few examples of nutrient-rich grains and seeds that can add texture, flavor, and a host of health benefits to meals. They provide the complex carbohydrates and fiber that help regulate blood sugar levels, preventing the energy spikes and crashes that can come from more refined options.

In this symphony of nutrient-dense foods, each ingredient plays a vital role, contributing its unique flavor, texture, and nutritional profile to the melody of a healthy diet. But beyond the individual nutrients, the magic lies in the way these foods come together, in meals that are not only nourishing but also deeply satisfying and enjoyable.

Eating for energy, especially for women over 50, is also about mindfulness and intention. It's about listening to the body's cues, understanding its needs, and responding with choices that nourish and invigorate. It's about enjoying the sensual pleasures of food, the joy of cooking and sharing meals, and the satisfaction of caring for one's body and soul.

This approach to eating is not about restriction or denial; it's about abundance and celebration. It's a way of eating that honors the body's wisdom, that cherishes the bounty of the earth, and that recognizes the power of food to heal, to comfort, and to energize. It's an invitation to explore, to experiment, and to discover the foods that make you feel alive, vibrant, and ready to embrace the beauty of life after 50.

As we embark on this journey of eating for energy, we do so

with the knowledge that food is more than just fuel. It's a way to connect with our bodies, with the world around us, and with the people we love. It's a pathway to vitality, a source of pleasure, and a celebration of life. In the rich tapestry of our days, nutrient-dense foods are the threads that weave together the picture of a life lived fully, joyously, and with abundant energy.

Understanding Macros and Micros

Navigating the world of nutrition, especially for women over 50, is akin to embarking on a profound journey of discovery, where the compass points towards understanding the intricate balance of macros (macronutrients) and micros (micronutrients). This exploration is not just about identifying what to eat; it's about uncovering the deeper narrative of how food fuels our bodies, supports our health, and energizes our lives. It's about crafting a diet that resonates with the rhythms of our bodies and the demands of our lives, providing a foundation for vitality, wellness, and joy.

At the heart of this narrative is the concept of macronutrients—the proteins, carbohydrates, and fats that serve as the primary building blocks of our diet and the main sources of energy for our bodies. Understanding the role and balance of these macronutrients is pivotal for women over 50, as it directly impacts energy levels, muscle maintenance, and overall health.

Proteins, the building blocks of life, play a crucial role in this balance. They're not just about muscle repair and growth; they're essential for a host of bodily functions, including the production of hormones and enzymes, and the maintenance of tissues. For women over 50, ensuring adequate protein intake is vital for preserving muscle mass, which naturally declines with age. However, it's not just the quantity of protein that matters but the quality. Emphasizing lean sources of protein, such as fish, poultry, legumes, and plant-based options, can provide the necessary amino acids without the added burden of saturated fats.

Carbohydrates, often maligned in the diet culture, are actually the body's preferred source of energy. They fuel our brains, our workouts, and our daily activities. Yet, the key lies in selecting the right kinds of carbohydrates. Whole grains, fruits, vegetables, and legumes offer a complex array of carbohydrates that are broken down slowly, providing a steady stream of energy and keeping blood sugar levels stable. This is particularly important for women over 50, as stable blood sugar levels are crucial for energy, mood regulation, and overall health.

Fats, the final piece of the macronutrient puzzle, have undergone a rehabilitation of sorts in the nutritional world. Once vilified, healthy fats are now celebrated for their numerous benefits, including supporting brain health, absorbing vitamins, and providing a concentrated source of energy. For women over 50, incorporating sources of healthy fats such as avocados, nuts, seeds, and olive oil can not only boost energy levels but also support hormonal balance and cardiovascular health.

Yet, the narrative of nutrition is not complete without the often-overlooked yet equally crucial micronutrients—vitamins, minerals, antioxidants, and phytonutrients that play supporting yet vital roles in our health. These powerful compounds support immune function, bone health, and cellular repair, and they are essential for converting food into usable energy. A diet rich in a variety of fruits, vegetables, whole grains, and lean proteins can provide a symphony of micronutrients that harmonize to support energy levels, prevent disease, and enhance well-being.

Understanding the interplay of macros and micros is akin to mastering the art of nutrition. It's about more than just the individual components; it's about how they work together to create a symphony of health. For women over 50, this understanding can empower choices that support vitality, from selecting nutrient-dense foods that offer a balance of macros and micros to understanding how these nutrients interact to fuel the body and spirit.

Hydration, often the unsung hero of nutrition, plays a pivotal role in this symphony. Water is essential for virtually every bodily function, including digestion, absorption, circulation, and temperature regulation. It's also crucial for transporting nutrients to cells and removing waste products. Adequate hydration can enhance energy levels, improve physical performance, and support cognitive function. For women over 50, paying attention to hydration is essential, as the sense of thirst may diminish with age, increasing the risk of dehydration.

Hydration: The Unsung Hero

In the vast landscape of nutrition and wellness, particularly for women over 50, hydration emerges not merely as a fundamental aspect but as an unsung hero, a vital element that sustains life, vitality, and energy. This narrative explores the profound significance of hydration, delving into its myriad benefits, challenges, and strategies, all aimed at fostering a deeper understanding and appreciation for the role of water in our lives.

Water, the elixir of life, serves as the medium through which the symphony of our bodily functions plays out. It is the canvas upon which our body's complex biochemical reactions are painted. For women over 50, staying hydrated is akin to maintaining the flow of life's river, ensuring that every cell, every organ, and every system operates in harmony. The importance of hydration transcends the simple act of quenching thirst; it is about nurturing the body's inner workings, enhancing vitality, and optimizing health.

At its core, hydration supports every facet of our physiological function. It is essential for the optimal performance of the cardiovascular system, facilitating the seamless transport of nutrients and oxygen to cells, and for the removal of waste products, a process akin to a river cleansing the landscape through which it flows. Moreover, water plays a pivotal role in regulating body temperature, a critical consideration for women navigating the hormonal fluctuations associated with menopause, which can affect thermoregulation and sweat production.

The brain, a marvel of nature's engineering, is particularly sensitive to the effects of hydration. Cognitive functions such as memory, attention, and mood are closely linked to hydration status. Even mild dehydration can cloud clarity, diminish concentration, and cast a shadow over one's emotional landscape. For women over 50, ensuring adequate hydration is not just about physical health; it's about maintaining the vibrancy of the mind and the spirit.

The journey towards maintaining hydration is, however, fraught with challenges. As we age, our body's natural thirst signals can become more muted, whispering rather than shouting, making it easy to overlook the need for water until dehydration has already begun to weave its subtle signs of fatigue, confusion, and physical discomfort. Recognizing and responding to these whispers before they become cries for help is a skill, a practice of mindful hydration that involves tuning in to the body's subtle cues and nurturing it with the life-giving essence of water.

The art of hydration extends beyond the simple act of drinking water. It involves a holistic approach to nutrition and lifestyle that recognizes the diverse sources of hydration—from the fruits and vegetables that grace our plates, offering not just nutrients but also their water content, to the herbal teas that warm our souls and soothe our spirits. It's about creating rituals around hydration, infusing the act of drinking water with intention and gratitude, transforming it from a mundane task into a nourishing practice.

For women over 50, the strategies for staying hydrated are as varied and individual as the women themselves. It may involve starting the day with a glass of water to awaken the body and signal the start of a new chapter. It might include carrying a water bottle as a constant companion, a tangible reminder of the need to sip regularly. It could involve tracking water intake to ensure that the goal of adequate hydration is not just an aspiration but a reality.

Yet, hydration is more than just a personal journey; it's a communal narrative that underscores the interconnectedness of all aspects of health. It's a conversation between friends, a shared goal within families, and a collective endeavor within communities. It's about championing the cause of hydration, not just for the individual but for the collective well-being.

In the grand tapestry of nutrition and wellness for women over 50, hydration stands as a cornerstone, a testament to the simple yet profound truth that water is life. This narrative of hydration is not just a chapter in the story of health; it is a golden thread that weaves through every aspect of our being, connecting us to our vitality, our energy, and our essence. It is a reminder that, in the journey of life, the act of staying hydrated is an act of self-love, a practice of nurturing the body and soul, and a celebration of the vibrant life that flows within us.

The Intermittent Diet Cookbook

Breakfasts to Break Your Fast Right

Recipe 1: Mediterranean Sunrise Bowl

- **P.T.:** 20 minutes
- **Ingr.:** 1 cup cooked quinoa, ½ avocado sliced, 2 poached eggs, ½ cup cherry tomatoes halved, ¼ cup crumbled feta cheese, 2 tbsp. pesto sauce, salt and pepper to taste, fresh basil for garnish.
- **Serves:** 2
- **M.C.:** Boiling and Poaching
- **Procedure:** Begin by dividing the cooked quinoa between two bowls. Top each bowl with sliced avocado, poached eggs, and halved cherry tomatoes. Sprinkle crumbled feta cheese over each. Drizzle with pesto sauce and season with salt and pepper. Garnish with fresh basil leaves before serving.
- **N.V.:** Rich in protein, healthy fats, and fiber. Provides essential vitamins and minerals.

Recipe 2: Spiced Pear Oatmeal

- **P.T.:** 15 minutes
- **Ingr.:** 1 cup steel-cut oats, 2 cups almond milk, 1 ripe pear (diced), 1 tsp cinnamon, ½ tsp nutmeg, 2 tbsp honey, ¼ cup walnuts (chopped).
- **Serves:** 2

- **M.C.:** Simmering
- **Procedure:** In a medium saucepan, bring almond milk to a boil. Add steel-cut oats and reduce heat to simmer. Stir in diced pear, cinnamon, and nutmeg. Cook for 10-12 minutes until oats are soft. Serve hot, topped with honey and chopped walnuts.
- **N.V.:** High in dietary fiber, heart-healthy omega-3 fatty acids, and antioxidants.

Recipe 3: Avocado Toast with Smoked Salmon

- **P.T.:** 10 minutes
- **Ingr.:** 2 slices of whole-grain bread, 1 ripe avocado, 4 oz smoked salmon, 1 tbsp lemon juice, 2 tsp capers, fresh dill for garnish, salt and pepper to taste.
- **Serves:** 2
- **M.C.:** Toasting
- **Procedure:** Toast the bread slices to your preferred crispness. Mash the avocado with lemon juice, salt, and pepper, and spread evenly on the toast. Top with smoked salmon, sprinkle with capers, and garnish with fresh dill.
- **N.V.:** Offers omega-3 fatty acids, protein, and essential vitamins.

Recipe 4: Tropical Smoothie Bowl

- **P.T.:** 10 minutes

- **Ingr.:** 1 frozen banana, ½ cup frozen mango chunks, ½ cup pineapple chunks, 1 cup coconut milk, 2 tbsp shredded coconut, 1 tbsp chia seeds, assorted toppings (kiwi slices, blueberries, granola).
- **Serves:** 1
- **M.C.:** Blending
- **Procedure:** Blend banana, mango, pineapple, and coconut milk until smooth. Pour into a bowl and top with shredded coconut, chia seeds, and your choice of toppings.
- **N.V.:** High in vitamin C, fiber, and healthy fats.

Recipe 5: Zucchini and Bell Pepper Frittata

- **P.T.:** 30 minutes
- **Ingr.:** 6 eggs, 1 zucchini (sliced), 1 bell pepper (diced), ¼ cup milk, ½ cup shredded cheese, salt and pepper to taste, 1 tbsp olive oil.
- **Serves:** 4
- **M.C.:** Baking
- **Procedure:** Preheat oven to 375°F (190°C). In a skillet, sauté zucchini and bell pepper in olive oil until soft. Whisk eggs, milk, salt, and pepper in a bowl. Add sautéed vegetables and cheese. Pour mixture into a greased baking dish. Bake for 20-25 minutes until set.
- **N.V.:** Rich in protein, vitamins A and C, and calcium.

Lunches That Fuel Your Afternoon

Recipe 1: Southwest Quinoa Salad

- **P.T.:** 25 minutes
- **Ingr.:** 1 cup quinoa, 2 cups water, 1 can black beans (drained and rinsed), 1 cup corn kernels (fresh or frozen), 1 red bell pepper (diced), 1 avocado (diced), 1/4 cup fresh cilantro (chopped), 1 lime (juice), 2 tablespoons olive oil, 1 teaspoon cumin, Salt and pepper to taste.
- **Serves:** 4
- **M.C.:** Boiling and Mixing
- **Procedure:**
  1. Rinse quinoa under cold water. In a medium saucepan, bring 2 cups of water to a boil. Add quinoa, reduce heat to low, cover, and simmer for 15 minutes or until water is absorbed. Remove from heat and let it stand covered for 5 minutes. Fluff with a fork and allow to cool.
  2. In a large bowl, combine cooled quinoa, black beans, corn, red bell pepper, and avocado.
  3. In a small bowl, whisk together lime juice, olive oil, cumin, salt, and pepper. Pour dressing over the quinoa mixture and toss to combine.
  4. Garnish with fresh cilantro before serving.

- **N.V.:** This salad is rich in plant-based protein from quinoa and black beans, providing essential amino acids. The avocado offers healthy monounsaturated fats, while the lime dressing adds a dose of vitamin C, enhancing iron absorption and boosting immunity.

Recipe 2: Thai Peanut Chicken Wrap

- **P.T.:** 20 minutes
- **Ingr.:** 2 cups shredded cooked chicken breast, 4 whole wheat wraps, 1 cup shredded purple cabbage, 1 carrot (julienned), 1/4 cup cilantro leaves, 1/4 cup crunchy peanut butter, 1 tablespoon soy sauce, 1 tablespoon lime juice, 1 teaspoon honey, 1/2 teaspoon grated ginger, 1 clove garlic (minced), Crushed peanuts for garnish.
- **Serves:** 4
- **M.C.:** Mixing and Wrapping
- **Procedure:**
  1. In a small bowl, whisk together peanut butter, soy sauce, lime juice, honey, ginger, and garlic until smooth. If the sauce is too thick, add a little water to reach the desired consistency.
  2. Lay out the wraps and spread each with the peanut sauce. Top with shredded chicken, purple cabbage, carrot, and cilantro leaves.
  3. Roll up the wraps tightly, cut in half, and sprinkle with crushed peanuts before serving.

- **N.V.:** Offers a good balance of lean protein from chicken, complex carbohydrates from the wrap, and healthy fats from peanut butter. The vegetables provide fiber and essential vitamins.

Recipe 3: Mediterranean Lentil Salad

- **P.T.:** 30 minutes
- **Ingr.:** 1 cup dry lentils, 1 cucumber (diced), 1 bell pepper (diced), 1/2 red onion (finely chopped), 1/2 cup crumbled feta cheese, 1/4 cup kalamata olives (halved), 1/4 cup extra virgin olive oil, 2 tablespoons red wine vinegar, 1 teaspoon dried oregano, Salt and pepper to taste.
- **Serves:** 4
- **M.C.:** Boiling and Mixing
- **Procedure:**
  1. Rinse lentils and cook in boiling water according to package instructions until tender. Drain and allow to cool.
  2. In a large bowl, combine cooled lentils, cucumber, bell pepper, red onion, feta cheese, and kalamata olives.
  3. In a small bowl, whisk together olive oil, red wine vinegar, oregano, salt, and pepper. Pour over the lentil mixture and toss to coat evenly.
  4. Chill in the refrigerator for about 20 minutes before serving to allow flavors to meld.

- **N.V.:** Lentils are a great source of plant-based protein and fiber. The salad is also high in healthy fats from olive oil and provides a good amount of vitamins and minerals from the fresh vegetables.

Recipe 4: Roasted Vegetable and Quinoa Bowl

- **P.T.:** 45 minutes
- **Ingr.:** 1 cup quinoa, 2 cups vegetable broth, 1 small sweet potato (cubed), 1 red bell pepper (sliced), 1 zucchini (sliced), 1 tablespoon olive oil, 1 teaspoon smoked paprika, Salt and pepper to taste, 1/4 cup toasted pumpkin seeds, 1 avocado (sliced).
- **Serves:** 4
- **M.C.:** Roasting and Boiling
- **Procedure:**
  1. Preheat oven to 425°F (220°C). Toss sweet potato, bell pepper, and zucchini with olive oil, smoked paprika, salt, and pepper. Spread on a baking sheet and roast for 25-30 minutes until tender.
  2. Meanwhile, rinse quinoa under cold water. Cook in vegetable broth according to package instructions until fluffy.
  3. Divide quinoa among bowls, top with roasted vegetables, pumpkin seeds, and sliced avocado.

- **N.V.:** Quinoa provides a complete protein source, while the vegetables offer fiber and essential nutrients. Avocado adds healthy fats, and pumpkin seeds contribute zinc and magnesium.

Recipe 5: Herb-Grilled Salmon with Avocado Salsa

- **P.T.:** 25 minutes
- **Ingr.:** 4 salmon fillets, 2 tablespoons olive oil, 1 teaspoon dried basil, 1 teaspoon dried oregano, Salt and pepper to taste, For the salsa: 1 ripe avocado (diced), 1/2 red onion (finely chopped), 1 tomato (diced), 1 lime (juice), 1/4 cup cilantro (chopped), Salt to taste.
- **Serves:** 4
- **M.C.:** Grilling
- **Procedure:**
  1. Preheat grill to medium-high heat. Brush salmon fillets with olive oil and season with basil, oregano, salt, and pepper.
  2. Grill salmon for about 4-5 minutes per side, or until cooked to your liking.
  3. In a bowl, mix together avocado, red onion, tomato, lime juice, cilantro, and salt to make the salsa.
  4. Serve grilled salmon topped with avocado salsa.

- **N.V.:** Salmon is an excellent source of omega-3 fatty acids, which are beneficial for heart health. The avocado salsa adds healthy fats, fiber, and a variety of vitamins and minerals.

Dinners to Satisfy and Nourish

Recipe 1: Lemon Herb Roasted Chicken

- **P.T.:** 1 hour 30 minutes
- **Ingr.:** 1 whole chicken (about 4 lbs), 2 lemons (1 juiced, 1 sliced), 4 cloves garlic (minced), 2 tablespoons olive oil, 1 tablespoon fresh rosemary (chopped), 1 tablespoon fresh thyme (chopped), Salt and pepper to taste, 1 lb baby potatoes (halved), 1 lb green beans (trimmed).
- **Serves:** 4
- **M.C.:** Roasting
- **Procedure:**
  1. Preheat your oven to 375°F (190°C). In a small bowl, mix olive oil, lemon juice, garlic, rosemary, thyme, salt, and pepper to create the marinade.
  2. Place the chicken in a roasting pan. Rub the marinade evenly over and inside the chicken. Stuff the chicken cavity with lemon slices.
  3. Surround the chicken with halved baby potatoes and sprinkle them with salt, pepper, and a

drizzle of olive oil.

4. Roast in the preheated oven for about 1 hour and 20 minutes, or until the chicken's internal temperature reaches 165°F (74°C). Add green beans to the roasting pan in the last 20 minutes of cooking.

5. Let the chicken rest for 10 minutes before carving. Serve with the roasted potatoes and green beans.

- **N.V.:** This meal is high in protein, essential for muscle repair and growth. The herbs and lemon provide vitamin C and antioxidants, while the baby potatoes offer a good source of potassium and fiber. Green beans add a low-calorie source of fiber and vitamins A, C, and K.

Recipe 2: Grilled Salmon with Mango Salsa

- **P.T.:** 30 minutes
- **Ingr.:** 4 salmon fillets (6 oz each), 1 ripe mango (diced), 1/2 red bell pepper (diced), 1/4 cup red onion (finely chopped), 1 jalapeño (seeded and minced), 2 tablespoons lime juice, 1 tablespoon olive oil, Salt and pepper to taste, 1/4 cup cilantro (chopped).
- **Serves:** 4
- **M.C.:** Grilling
- **Procedure:**
    1. Preheat grill to medium-high heat. Season

salmon fillets with salt, pepper, and a light brush of olive oil.

2. Grill salmon, skin-side down, for about 5-7 minutes. Flip carefully and continue grilling until cooked through, about 3-5 minutes more.

3. In a bowl, mix mango, red bell pepper, red onion, jalapeño, lime juice, and cilantro. Season with salt and pepper.

4. Serve grilled salmon topped with mango salsa.

- **N.V.:** Salmon is rich in omega-3 fatty acids, beneficial for heart health. The mango salsa provides a good source of vitamins A and C, fiber, and antioxidants.

Recipe 3: Vegetable Stir-Fry with Tofu

- **P.T.:** 25 minutes
- **Ingr.:** 1 block firm tofu (pressed and cubed), 2 cups broccoli florets, 1 red bell pepper (sliced), 1 cup snap peas, 1 carrot (julienned), 2 tablespoons soy sauce, 1 tablespoon sesame oil, 1 teaspoon ginger (grated), 2 cloves garlic (minced), 1 tablespoon cornstarch, 1/4 cup water, Sesame seeds for garnish.
- **Serves:** 4
- **M.C.:** Stir-frying
- **Procedure:**

1. Heat sesame oil in a large pan or wok over medium-high heat. Add tofu cubes and stir-fry until golden brown. Remove and set aside.

2. In the same pan, add broccoli, bell pepper, snap peas, and carrot. Stir-fry for about 5 minutes.

3. Mix soy sauce, ginger, garlic, cornstarch, and water in a small bowl. Pour over the vegetables, add tofu back to the pan, and cook until the sauce thickens.

4. Sprinkle with sesame seeds before serving.

- **N.V.:** High in protein from tofu. The vegetables provide a wealth of nutrients, including vitamins C and K, potassium, and fiber.

Recipe 4: Butternut Squash Risotto

- **P.T.:** 45 minutes
- **Ingr.:** 1 butternut squash (peeled and cubed), 1 tablespoon olive oil, 4 cups vegetable broth, 1 onion (finely chopped), 1 cup Arborio rice, 1/2 cup dry white wine, 1/4 cup grated Parmesan cheese, Salt and pepper to taste, Fresh sage for garnish.
- **Serves:** 4
- **M.C.:** Sautéing and Simmering
- **Procedure:**

1. Roast butternut squash with olive oil in a 400°F oven for 25 minutes until tender.

2. In a saucepan, heat broth over low heat. In another pan, sauté onion until translucent, add rice, and toast for 2 minutes. Deglaze with white wine.

3. Add broth one ladle at a time, stirring until absorbed before adding more. Halfway through, add roasted squash.

4. Once rice is creamy and cooked, stir in Parmesan. Season with salt and pepper, and garnish with sage.

- **N.V.:** A good source of complex carbohydrates and fiber from the rice and squash. The cheese adds calcium and protein.

Recipe 5: Moroccan Chickpea Stew

- **P.T.:** 40 minutes
- **Ingr.:** 2 cans chickpeas (drained and rinsed), 1 onion (chopped), 2 carrots (diced), 2 celery stalks (diced), 1 can diced tomatoes, 4 cups vegetable broth, 1 teaspoon cumin, 1/2 teaspoon cinnamon, 1/2 teaspoon paprika, 1/4 teaspoon cayenne pepper, Salt and pepper to taste, 2 tablespoons olive oil, Fresh cilantro for garnish.
- **Serves:** 4
- **M.C.:** Sautéing and Simmering
- **Procedure:**

1. Heat olive oil in a large pot over medium heat. Add onion, carrots, and celery. Cook until softened.

2. Stir in spices, then add chickpeas, diced tomatoes, and vegetable broth. Bring to a boil, then reduce heat and simmer for 30 minutes.

3. Season with salt and pepper. Serve hot, garnished with fresh cilantro.

- **N.V.:** Chickpeas are a great source of plant-based protein and fiber. The spices offer anti-inflammatory benefits, and the vegetables add essential vitamins and minerals.

Snacks and Beverages: Your IF Allies

Recipe 1: Cucumber Mint Infusion

- **P.T.:** 5 minutes (+ 1 hour chilling time)
- **Ingr.:** 1 large cucumber (thinly sliced), 10 fresh mint leaves, 2 quarts of water, Ice cubes for serving, Optional: 1 lime (sliced) for added flavor.
- **Serves:** 8
- **M.C.:** Infusing
- **Procedure:**
    1. In a large pitcher, combine cucumber slices, mint leaves, and lime slices if using.
    2. Fill the pitcher with water. Stir gently to combine.
    3. Refrigerate for at least 1 hour to allow the flavors to infuse. The longer it sits, the more pronounced the flavors.
    4. Serve over ice in glasses. Garnish with additional mint leaves or cucumber slices if desired.

- **N.V.:** Virtually calorie-free. Cucumbers and mint offer refreshing and hydrating properties, making this infusion an excellent ally for maintaining hydration and aiding digestion during fasting periods.

Recipe 2: Almond Butter Energy Balls

- **P.T.:** 15 minutes (plus 30 minutes chilling time)
- **Ingr.:** 1 cup rolled oats, 1/2 cup almond butter, 1/4 cup honey or maple syrup, 1/4 cup chia seeds, 1/2 cup dark chocolate chips, 1 teaspoon vanilla extract, A pinch of salt.
- **Serves:** 12 balls
- **M.C.:** Mixing
- **Procedure:**
  1. In a large bowl, mix together rolled oats, almond butter, honey or maple syrup, chia seeds, dark chocolate chips, vanilla extract, and a pinch of salt until well combined.
  2. Roll the mixture into small balls, about 1 inch in diameter, and place them on a baking sheet lined with parchment paper.
  3. Chill in the refrigerator for at least 30 minutes to set.
  4. Store in an airtight container in the refrigerator.
- **N.V.:** Rich in dietary fiber from oats and chia seeds, healthy fats from almond butter, and antioxidants from dark chocolate. Provides a good balance of

macronutrients for sustained energy.

Recipe 3: Spicy Roasted Chickpeas

- **P.T.:** 40 minutes
- **Ingr.:** 2 cans chickpeas (drained, rinsed, and patted dry), 2 tablespoons olive oil, 1/2 teaspoon smoked paprika, 1/2 teaspoon garlic powder, 1/4 teaspoon cayenne pepper, Salt to taste.
- **Serves:** 4
- **M.C.:** Roasting
- **Procedure:**
  1. Preheat the oven to 400°F (200°C).
  2. Toss chickpeas with olive oil, smoked paprika, garlic powder, cayenne pepper, and salt in a bowl.
  3. Spread chickpeas on a baking sheet in a single layer.
  4. Roast for 30-35 minutes, stirring occasionally, until crispy and golden.
  5. Let cool before serving.
- **N.V.:** Chickpeas are a great source of plant-based protein and fiber, making them an ideal snack for energy and satiety. The spices add flavor without adding calories.

Recipe 4: Green Tea & Honey Iced Tea

- **P.T.:** 10 minutes (+ chilling time)
- **Ingr.:** 4 green tea bags, 4 cups boiling water, 2

tablespoons honey, Ice cubes, Fresh mint or lemon slices for garnish.

- **Serves:** 4
- **M.C.:** Brewing and Chilling
- **Procedure:**
    1. Steep green tea bags in boiling water for 3-5 minutes, depending on desired strength.
    2. Remove tea bags and stir in honey until dissolved.
    3. Let the tea cool to room temperature, then refrigerate until chilled.
    4. Serve over ice, garnished with fresh mint or lemon slices.
- **N.V.:** Green tea is rich in antioxidants, supporting overall health. Honey provides a natural source of energy and sweetness.

Recipe 5: Avocado & Tomato Crackers

- **P.T.:** 10 minutes
- **Ingr.:** Whole-grain crackers, 1 ripe avocado, 1 small tomato (sliced), Salt and pepper to taste, Crushed red pepper flakes (optional).
- **Serves:** 2-3
- **M.C.:** Assembling
- **Procedure:**
    1. Mash the avocado in a small bowl. Season with salt and pepper.

2. Spread the mashed avocado evenly on whole-grain crackers.

3. Top each cracker with a slice of tomato. Sprinkle with crushed red pepper flakes if desired.

- **N.V.:** Provides healthy fats from avocado, fiber from whole-grain crackers, and vitamins from tomatoes. A balanced snack to support energy levels.

Special Dietary Considerations

Adapting Recipes for Food Sensitivities

Recipe 1: Gluten-Free Quinoa Tabbouleh

- **P.T.:** 20 minutes
- **Ingr.:** 1 cup quinoa (rinsed), 2 cups water, 1 cucumber (diced), 2 tomatoes (diced), 1/4 cup fresh parsley (chopped), 1/4 cup fresh mint (chopped), 1/4 cup lemon juice, 2 tablespoons olive oil, Salt and pepper to taste.
- **Serves:** 4
- **M.C.:** Boiling and Mixing
- **Procedure:**
  1. In a medium saucepan, bring water to a boil. Add quinoa, reduce heat to low, cover, and simmer for 15 minutes, or until water is absorbed. Remove from heat and let stand for 5 minutes, then fluff with a fork and allow to cool.
  2. In a large bowl, combine the cooled quinoa, diced cucumber, tomatoes, chopped parsley, and mint.
  3. In a small bowl, whisk together lemon juice, olive oil, salt, and pepper. Pour over the quinoa mixture and toss to combine thoroughly.

4. Refrigerate for at least 1 hour before serving to allow flavors to meld.

- **N.V.:** Quinoa provides a high-protein, gluten-free alternative to bulgur wheat traditionally used in tabbouleh, making this recipe suitable for those with gluten sensitivities. This dish is also rich in vitamins A and C from the vegetables and herbs, and provides healthy fats from olive oil.

Recipe 2: Dairy-Free Creamy Mushroom Soup

- **P.T.:** 30 minutes
- **Ingr.:** 2 tablespoons olive oil, 1 onion (chopped), 2 cloves garlic (minced), 1 lb mushrooms (sliced), 4 cups vegetable broth, 1 cup coconut cream, 1 tablespoon fresh thyme (chopped), Salt and pepper to taste.
- **Serves:** 4
- **M.C.:** Sautéing and Simmering
- **Procedure:**
    1. Heat olive oil in a large pot over medium heat. Add onion and garlic, sautéing until soft.
    2. Add mushrooms and thyme, cooking until mushrooms are browned.
    3. Pour in vegetable broth, bringing to a boil. Reduce heat and simmer for 20 minutes.
    4. Stir in coconut cream and season with salt and pepper. Use an immersion blender to puree the soup until smooth.

- **N.V.:** This soup is a comforting, dairy-free option rich in umami from mushrooms. Coconut cream provides a creamy texture without dairy, suitable for lactose intolerance.

Recipe 3: Nut-Free Pesto Pasta

- **P.T.:** 20 minutes
- **Ingr.:** 1 lb gluten-free pasta, 2 cups fresh basil leaves, 1/2 cup olive oil, 1/2 cup sunflower seeds (toasted), 2 cloves garlic, 1/2 cup grated parmesan cheese (or nutritional yeast for dairy-free), Salt and pepper to taste.
- **Serves:** 4
- **M.C.:** Boiling and Blending
- **Procedure:**
  1. Cook pasta according to package instructions. Drain and set aside.
  2. In a food processor, combine basil, olive oil, sunflower seeds, garlic, and parmesan cheese (or nutritional yeast). Process until smooth.
  3. Toss the pesto with the cooked pasta, seasoning with salt and pepper.
- **N.V.:** Offers a nut-free alternative to traditional pesto, using sunflower seeds. It's rich in healthy fats from olive oil and provides a good source of protein and fiber from gluten-free pasta.

Recipe 4: Soy-Free Teriyaki Chicken

- **P.T.:** 45 minutes
- **Ingr.:** 4 chicken breasts, For the marinade: 1/2 cup coconut aminos, 1/4 cup honey, 2 cloves garlic (minced), 1 teaspoon ginger (grated), 1 tablespoon apple cider vinegar, Salt and pepper to taste, Sesame seeds and sliced green onions for garnish.
- **Serves:** 4
- **M.C.:** Marinating and Baking
- **Procedure:**
    1. Whisk together coconut aminos, honey, garlic, ginger, apple cider vinegar, salt, and pepper. Marinate chicken breasts for at least 30 minutes.
    2. Preheat oven to 375°F. Place marinated chicken in a baking dish, pouring over any remaining marinade.
    3. Bake for 25-30 minutes, or until chicken is cooked through.
    4. Garnish with sesame seeds and green onions before serving.
- **N.V.:** Utilizes coconut aminos as a soy-free alternative to traditional soy sauce, making this dish suitable for those avoiding soy. Offers a good source of protein and is seasoned with natural ingredients for flavor.

Recipe 5: Gluten-Free Almond Flour Chocolate Chip Cookies

- **P.T.:** 25 minutes

- **Ingr.:** 2 cups almond flour, 1/2 cup coconut oil (melted), 1/2 cup maple syrup, 1 teaspoon vanilla extract, 1/2 teaspoon baking soda, A pinch of salt, 1/2 cup dark chocolate chips (dairy-free if necessary).
- **Serves:** 12 cookies
- **M.C.:** Baking
- **Procedure:**
  1. Preheat the oven to 350°F and line a baking sheet with parchment paper.
  2. In a bowl, mix together almond flour, baking soda, and salt. Stir in melted coconut oil, maple syrup, and vanilla extract until a dough forms.
  3. Fold in chocolate chips. Drop tablespoonfuls of dough onto the prepared baking sheet.
  4. Bake for 10-12 minutes, or until edges are golden. Let cool on the baking sheet.
- **N.V.:** These cookies are a delightful treat for those with gluten sensitivity, using almond flour as a gluten-free base. They're sweetened naturally with maple syrup and include healthy fats from coconut oil.

Vegetarian and Vegan Options

Recipe 1: Vegan Thai Coconut Curry

- **P.T.:** 30 minutes

- **Ingr.:** 1 tbsp coconut oil, 1 onion (diced), 2 cloves garlic (minced), 1 tbsp ginger (grated), 1 red bell pepper (sliced), 1 zucchini (sliced), 1 carrot (julienned), 1 cup broccoli florets, 2 tbsp red curry paste, 1 can (14 oz) coconut milk, 1 tbsp soy sauce (or tamari for GF option), 1 tsp maple syrup, Juice of 1 lime, Salt to taste, Fresh cilantro and sliced chili for garnish, Cooked rice for serving.
- **Serves:** 4
- **M.C.:** Sautéing and Simmering
- **Procedure:**
  1. Heat coconut oil in a large skillet over medium heat. Add onion, garlic, and ginger, sautéing until onion is translucent.
  2. Stir in bell pepper, zucchini, carrot, and broccoli, cooking until slightly softened.
  3. Add curry paste, stirring until vegetables are coated. Pour in coconut milk, soy sauce, maple syrup, and lime juice. Simmer for 10-15 minutes.
  4. Season with salt, adjust flavors as needed. Serve over rice, garnished with cilantro and chili.
- **N.V.:** Rich in vitamins and minerals from the vegetables, healthy fats from coconut milk, and protein from the addition of tofu or chickpeas if desired.

Recipe 2: Quinoa Stuffed Bell Peppers

- **P.T.:** 45 minutes

- **Ingr.:** 4 large bell peppers (halved and seeded), 1 cup quinoa (cooked), 1 can (15 oz) black beans (rinsed and drained), 1 cup corn kernels, 1/2 cup tomato sauce, 1 tsp cumin, 1 tsp paprika, Salt and pepper to taste, 1/2 cup shredded vegan cheese, Fresh cilantro for garnish.
- **Serves:** 4
- **M.C.:** Baking
- **Procedure:**
  1. Preheat oven to 375°F (190°C). Place bell pepper halves in a baking dish, cut-side up.
  2. In a bowl, mix quinoa, black beans, corn, tomato sauce, cumin, paprika, salt, and pepper.
  3. Fill each bell pepper half with the quinoa mixture. Top with vegan cheese.
  4. Cover with foil and bake for 30 minutes. Uncover and bake for an additional 10 minutes.
  5. Garnish with fresh cilantro before serving.
- **N.V.:** Offers a balanced meal with protein from quinoa and black beans, fiber from vegetables, and calcium from vegan cheese.

Recipe 3: Vegan Mushroom Stroganoff

- **P.T.:** 25 minutes
- **Ingr.:** 1 tbsp olive oil, 1 onion (chopped), 2 cloves garlic (minced), 1 lb mushrooms (sliced), 2 tbsp all-purpose flour (use GF if needed), 2 cups vegetable broth, 1 tbsp soy sauce (or tamari for GF), 1 tsp thyme, 1/2 cup vegan

sour cream, Salt and pepper to taste, Cooked pasta for serving.

- **Serves:** 4
- **M.C.:** Sautéing and Boiling
- **Procedure:**
  1. Heat oil in a large skillet over medium heat. Add onion and garlic, cooking until softened.
  2. Add mushrooms, sauté until browned. Sprinkle with flour, stir to coat.
  3. Gradually add broth and soy sauce, bring to a simmer. Cook until thickened.
  4. Stir in vegan sour cream and thyme. Season with salt and pepper.
  5. Serve over cooked pasta, garnished with fresh herbs.
- **N.V.:** A comforting, creamy dish high in protein from mushrooms and enriched with B vitamins from nutritional yeast if added to the sauce.

Recipe 4: Lentil and Walnut Tacos

- **P.T.:** 30 minutes
- **Ingr.:** 1 cup green lentils (cooked), 1/2 cup walnuts (chopped), 1 tbsp olive oil, 1 onion (diced), 2 cloves garlic (minced), 2 tsp chili powder, 1 tsp cumin, Salt and pepper to taste, Taco shells, Toppings: lettuce, tomato, avocado, vegan cheese, lime wedges.
- **Serves:** 4

- **M.C.:** Sautéing
- **Procedure:**
  1. Heat oil in a pan over medium heat. Add onion and garlic, cook until translucent.
  2. Add lentils, walnuts, chili powder, cumin, salt, and pepper. Cook for 5-7 minutes.
  3. Warm taco shells according to package instructions.
  4. Assemble tacos by filling shells with the lentil mixture. Top with lettuce, tomato, avocado, and vegan cheese.
  5. Serve with lime wedges on the side.
- **N.V.:** Lentils and walnuts provide a hearty, meaty texture and are excellent sources of protein and omega-3 fatty acids.

Recipe 5: Creamy Avocado Pasta

- **P.T.:** 15 minutes
- **Ingr.:** 2 ripe avocados, 2 cloves garlic, Juice of 1 lemon, 1/4 cup olive oil, Salt and pepper to taste, 1/2 cup fresh basil leaves, 12 oz pasta (gluten-free if needed), Cherry tomatoes for garnish.
- **Serves:** 4
- **M.C.:** Boiling and Blending
- **Procedure:**
  1. Cook pasta according to package directions. Drain, reserving some pasta water.

2. While pasta cooks, blend avocados, garlic, lemon juice, olive oil, salt, pepper, and basil in a food processor until smooth.

3. Toss pasta with the avocado sauce, adding pasta water as needed to achieve desired consistency.

4. Serve garnished with cherry tomatoes and additional basil.

- **N.V.:** The sauce provides healthy fats from avocado and olive oil, while the whole-grain or gluten-free pasta offers fiber. A light yet satisfying meal.

Balancing Indulgences and Healthy Eating

Recipe 1: Dark Chocolate Avocado Mousse

- **P.T.:** 15 minutes (plus chilling)
- **Ingr.:** 2 ripe avocados, peeled and pitted; 1/4 cup unsweetened cocoa powder; 1/4 cup high-quality dark chocolate, melted; 1/4 cup maple syrup; 1 teaspoon vanilla extract; A pinch of salt; Fresh berries for topping.
- **Serves:** 4
- **M.C.:** Blending
- **Procedure:**
  1. Combine avocados, cocoa powder, melted dark chocolate, maple syrup, vanilla extract, and a pinch of salt in a food processor.

2. Blend until smooth and creamy, scraping down the sides as necessary.

3. Divide the mousse into serving dishes and refrigerate for at least an hour.

4. Serve chilled, topped with fresh berries.

- **N.V.:** Rich in healthy fats from avocado and antioxidants from dark chocolate. A satisfying dessert that's both indulgent and nutrient-dense.

Recipe 2: Zesty Lemon Baked Salmon

- **P.T.:** 25 minutes
- **Ingr.:** 4 salmon fillets (6 oz each); 2 lemons, 1 sliced and 1 juiced; 2 tablespoons olive oil; 1 tablespoon honey; 1 garlic clove, minced; 1 teaspoon dried dill; Salt and pepper to taste; Asparagus spears as a side.
- **Serves:** 4
- **M.C.:** Baking
- **Procedure:**

  1. Preheat the oven to 375°F (190°C). Place salmon fillets in a baking dish.

  2. Whisk together lemon juice, olive oil, honey, minced garlic, dill, salt, and pepper. Pour over salmon.

  3. Arrange lemon slices and asparagus around the salmon.

  4. Bake for 15-20 minutes, until salmon is cooked through and asparagus is tender.

- **N.V.:** Salmon is a great source of omega-3 fatty acids, protein, and vitamin D. Asparagus adds fiber, vitamins A, C, E, and K.

Recipe 3: Quinoa and Black Bean Stuffed Peppers

- **P.T.:** 1 hour
- **Ingr.:** 4 large bell peppers, halved and seeded; 1 cup quinoa, cooked; 1 can black beans, drained and rinsed; 1 cup corn kernels; 1/2 cup tomato sauce; 1 teaspoon cumin; 1/2 teaspoon smoked paprika; Salt and pepper to taste; 1/2 cup shredded cheese (optional).
- **Serves:** 4
- **M.C.:** Baking
- **Procedure:**
    1. Preheat oven to 350°F (175°C). Arrange bell pepper halves in a baking dish.
    2. In a bowl, mix quinoa, black beans, corn, tomato sauce, cumin, smoked paprika, salt, and pepper.
    3. Fill each bell pepper half with the quinoa mixture. Top with cheese if using.
    4. Cover with foil and bake for 30 minutes. Uncover and bake for another 10 minutes, until peppers are tender.
- **N.V.:** A fiber-rich meal with a good balance of complex carbohydrates, protein, and vitamins.

Recipe 4: Spinach and Feta Turkey Burgers

- **P.T.:** 30 minutes

- **Ingr.:** 1 lb ground turkey; 2 cups fresh spinach, chopped; 1/2 cup feta cheese, crumbled; 1 egg, beaten; 2 cloves garlic, minced; 1 teaspoon oregano; Salt and pepper to taste; Whole-grain buns for serving.
- **Serves:** 4
- **M.C.:** Grilling
- **Procedure:**
  1. In a large bowl, mix together ground turkey, spinach, feta, egg, garlic, oregano, salt, and pepper.
  2. Form the mixture into 4 patties.
  3. Grill over medium heat for 5-7 minutes per side, until fully cooked.
  4. Serve on whole-grain buns with your choice of toppings.
- **N.V.:** Offers lean protein from turkey, calcium from feta, and iron and vitamins from spinach.

Recipe 5: Sweet Potato and Chickpea Buddha Bowl

- **P.T.:** 45 minutes
- **Ingr.:** 2 large sweet potatoes, cubed; 1 can chickpeas, drained, rinsed, and patted dry; 2 tablespoons olive oil; 1 teaspoon each of cumin, coriander, and smoked paprika; Salt and pepper to taste; 2 cups spinach leaves; 1 avocado, sliced; 1/4 cup tahini; Juice of 1 lemon; 1 garlic clove, minced.
- **Serves:** 4

- **M.C.:** Roasting
- **Procedure:**
  1. Preheat oven to 425°F (220°C). Toss sweet potatoes and chickpeas with olive oil, cumin, coriander, smoked paprika, salt, and pepper.
  2. Spread on a baking sheet and roast for 30-35 minutes, until sweet potatoes are tender.
  3. Arrange spinach leaves in bowls. Top with roasted sweet potatoes, chickpeas, and avocado slices.
  4. Whisk together tahini, lemon juice, garlic, and water (as needed) for the dressing. Drizzle over each bowl.
- **N.V.:** A nutrient-dense meal providing healthy fats, protein, fiber, and a range of vitamins and minerals from the diverse ingredients.

Part VI: Beyond the Diet

The Role of Sleep and Recovery

Sleep's Impact on Weight and Well-being

The narrative of sleep's influence on weight management is a tale as old as time, yet it's only in recent years that we've begun to decode its complexities. At the heart of this relationship lies the delicate balance of two key hormones: ghrelin and leptin. Ghrelin, often dubbed the "hunger hormone," signals the brain to encourage eating. Leptin, on the other hand, communicates satiety, telling us when it's time to stop eating. Sleep deprivation skews the balance of these hormones, elevating ghrelin levels while diminishing leptin, leading to increased hunger and appetite. This hormonal imbalance, often compounded by the body's craving for high-calorie, carbohydrate-rich foods for quick energy, can result in weight gain, setting the stage for a challenging cycle of sleep disruption and dietary excess.

Moreover, sleep's role in metabolism casts a long shadow over our body's ability to manage weight. During the deep stages of rest, the body enters a state of repair, where cells rejuvenate, and energy is conserved and redirected towards processing nutrients and stabilizing blood sugar levels. Insufficient sleep hampers this process, leading to poor insulin regulation, which can spiral into weight gain or, in severe cases, contribute to the development of type 2 diabetes.

But the impact of sleep extends beyond the confines of physical health, meandering into the realms of mental and emotional well-being. A lack of restorative sleep can fray the edges of our emotional resilience, making us more susceptible to stress and anxiety. This heightened emotional state can trigger comfort eating, further complicating the relationship between sleep and weight. Additionally, the fog of fatigue that envelops a sleep-deprived mind dulls cognitive function, impeding decision-making and willpower, which are crucial for maintaining a healthy lifestyle and making balanced dietary choices.

The symphony of sleep also plays a vital role in physical recovery and performance. For those engaged in regular exercise as part of a weight management or well-being program, sleep is the unsung hero that facilitates muscle repair, strength building, and recovery. Growth hormone, released during deep sleep, orchestrates this process, aiding in the development of lean muscle mass, which in turn supports a healthy metabolism.

Understanding sleep's pivotal role in weight and well-being illuminates the necessity of nurturing our sleep environment and habits. It beckons us to prioritize rest as much as we do diet and exercise, recognizing that sleep is not merely a passive state but an active, restorative process that shapes our health, well-being, and quality of life.

In this light, the quest for better sleep becomes a cornerstone of holistic health. It challenges us to dismantle the barriers to restful nights, from the blue light of screens that disrupt our circadian rhythms to the stress and anxieties that keep us tossing and turning. It invites us to create rituals that signal the body and mind to unwind, to foster environments that cradle us into sleep, and to embrace practices that soothe the soul and quiet the mind.

Thus, the journey towards understanding and improving sleep is not a solitary endeavor but a collective voyage that requires us to rethink our relationship with the night, to respect the rhythms of our bodies, and to revere the sanctity of sleep. In doing so, we unlock the door to better health, improved weight management, and a well-being that radiates from the inside out, illuminating the path to a life lived in harmony with the natural world and with ourselves.

Delving deeper into the narrative of sleep's profound influence on weight management and overall well-being, we uncover a multifaceted story that intertwines our biological, psychological, and environmental threads. This intricate relationship underscores the fundamental truth that our bodies are not mere machines that can be fueled and refueled without regard for the quality of rest and repair they receive. Instead, they are complex organisms that thrive on balance, harmony, and the rhythmic dance between activity and rest.

The hormonal interplay between ghrelin and leptin serves as a prime example of this balance. Modern lifestyles, characterized by late-night screen time, irregular sleeping patterns, and the ever-present lure of calorie-dense, nutrient-poor foods, have thrown this delicate balance into disarray. The increase in ghrelin and decrease in leptin levels due to sleep deprivation not only trigger physical hunger but also amplify the emotional need for comfort through food, leading individuals down a path of late-night snacking and overeating that further disrupts sleep quality. It's a cyclical battle, where each night of insufficient rest compounds the body's craving for quick energy fixes, perpetuating a cycle of weight gain and sleep disturbances.

This cycle is further complicated by the body's metabolic processes during sleep. The state of rest is not simply a pause in our daily activities but a critical period for metabolic health. It's when the body performs its maintenance, repairing tissues, synthesizing hormones, and processing the day's nutrient intake. Sleep deprivation cuts this process short, impairing glucose metabolism and insulin sensitivity, thereby increasing the risk of obesity and diabetes. It's akin to running a factory non-stop without allowing time for machinery maintenance, eventually leading to breakdowns and decreased efficiency.

The psychological ramifications of sleep deprivation extend this narrative into the realm of mental and emotional health.

The impact on cognitive functions, including decision-making and impulse control, directly affects dietary choices, often leading to a preference for high-sugar, high-fat foods. Moreover, the emotional toll of chronic fatigue, characterized by increased irritability, anxiety, and stress, can lead to emotional eating as a coping mechanism, further entrenching the cycle of weight gain and poor sleep.

Engaging in regular physical activity is widely advocated as a means to improve both sleep quality and weight management. However, without adequate rest, the body cannot fully benefit from exercise. The release of growth hormone during deep sleep phases is crucial for muscle repair and building, which in turn supports a more active metabolism. Neglecting sleep undermines the benefits of exercise, diminishing returns on physical health efforts and further complicating weight management challenges.

Recognizing the importance of sleep requires a holistic approach to health and well-being, one that values rest as much as diet and exercise. Creating a sleep-conducive environment, free from the disruptions of technology and stress, alongside establishing pre-sleep rituals that promote relaxation, can significantly enhance the quality of rest. Whether it's through reducing caffeine intake in the afternoon, practicing mindfulness or meditation before bed, or ensuring the sleep environment is dark, cool, and quiet, these strategies collectively support the body's natural sleep-wake cycle.

Embracing the quest for better sleep is an invitation to transform our relationship with the night, to see it not as a time of inactivity or lost productivity but as a vital component of a life well-lived. It's a commitment to honoring the body's need for rest, to nurturing the mind's need for tranquility, and to fostering a lifestyle that places well-being at its core.

In navigating this journey, we not only enhance our capacity for weight management but also enrich our lives with improved mental clarity, emotional resilience, and overall vitality. The path to better health and well-being, illuminated by the glow of restful nights and balanced days, becomes a journey of rediscovery, where each step taken in harmony with our natural rhythms brings us closer to our true selves and the life we aspire to live.

Creating a Restorative Sleep Environment

Creating a restorative sleep environment is an art that intertwines elements of physical comfort, sensory reduction, and psychological peace to foster deep, rejuvenating sleep. This holistic approach to designing our nightly sanctuaries is more than a mere backdrop for rest; it's a foundational pillar for health, weight management, and overall well-being.

The journey to crafting such an environment begins with understanding the profound impact of our surroundings on sleep quality. Every detail, from the texture of our bedding to the quality of air, plays a pivotal role in either inviting restfulness or perpetuating restlessness.

Central to our sleep environment is the interplay between light and darkness, a crucial factor given its direct influence on our circadian rhythms. Melatonin, often referred to as the hormone of darkness, signals to our bodies when it's time to rest. Exposure to bright and particularly blue light from screens can severely disrupt this natural cycle, tricking our brains into a state of alertness well into the night. Thus, cultivating darkness in our sleep spaces becomes paramount. This can be achieved through the use of blackout curtains or sleep masks, alongside a curfew on screen time to protect the sanctity of our internal clocks.

Noise, or rather the absence of it, is another cornerstone of a restorative sleep environment. The intrusion of sound, whether from urban clamor or household bustle, can fragment our sleep cycles, leaving us hovering in the lighter stages of rest. The solution lies in the embrace of silence or the strategic use of white noise or soothing sounds to mask disruptive noises. Sound machines or apps that simulate the rhythmic, gentle sounds of nature can serve as a cocoon of calm, enveloping us in an auditory landscape conducive to deep sleep.

Physical comfort, from the firmness of our mattresses to the softness of our sheets, paints the canvas of our sleep experience. The tactile relationship we share with our sleep surfaces can be deeply personal, with individual preferences guiding the choice of bedding materials that support the body's natural alignment and breathability. Investing in high-quality, natural fibers for bedding and selecting a mattress that complements one's sleep style can transform a mere bed into a cradle of comfort and restoration.

The quality of air in our sleep environment often goes unnoticed, yet its impact on sleep quality is profound. A room that's too dry or laden with allergens can disturb sleep through discomfort and respiratory issues. Maintaining a clean, well-ventilated room with the aid of air purifiers or humidifiers can ensure the air we breathe throughout the night supports, rather than detracts from, our health.

Color, often celebrated for its emotional and psychological influence, can transform the aesthetic of a bedroom into a sanctuary of sleep. Soft, soothing colors like muted blues, greens, and earth tones can lower heart rate and blood pressure, easing the transition into sleep. The visual serenity of the room, paired with personal touches that spark joy and relaxation, can significantly enhance the sleep experience.

Beyond the physical environment, preparing oneself for sleep through pre-sleep rituals can signal the body and mind to wind down. Whether it's a warm bath, reading by soft light, or gentle stretching, these activities can bridge the gap between the hustle of the day and the peace of the night, fostering a mental environment ready for rest.

Finally, the consistency of our sleep environment and routines cannot be overstated. Our bodies thrive on predictability, with regular sleep and wake times reinforcing our natural circadian rhythms. This commitment to continuity, both in the environment we craft and the routines we follow, cements the foundation for restorative sleep.

In curating a restorative sleep environment, we do more than just decorate a room; we sculpt a retreat that honors our need for rest, recovery, and rejuvenation. It's a testament to the understanding that sleep is not a luxury, but a necessity, deserving of intention and respect. Through this lens, the quest for better sleep becomes an integral part of our journey toward health, weight management, and well-being, illuminating the path to a life lived in harmony with our natural rhythms and needs.

Relaxation Techniques for Better Sleep

In the realm of sleep, the mind is both a gatekeeper and a wanderer, capable of transporting us to realms of deep rest or holding us back with tendrils of stress and anxiety. Mindfulness meditation emerges as a powerful tool in this context, offering a pathway to mental stillness and sleep readiness. This practice involves focusing on the breath, allowing thoughts to come and go without attachment, creating a state of calm that paves the way for sleep. By dedicating time each night to mindfulness, perhaps through guided meditations or breathing exercises, individuals can train their minds to transition smoothly into sleep, enhancing both the speed of falling asleep and the quality of rest achieved.

Yoga, with its harmonious blend of physical postures, controlled breathing, and meditation, serves as a bridge to better sleep. Engaging in a gentle yoga sequence before bed can release physical tension, calm the nervous system, and focus the mind, all of which contribute to a state conducive to sleep. Poses such as forward folds, gentle twists, and legs-up-the-wall can be particularly beneficial, promoting relaxation and circulation. Integrating yoga into the evening routine is not just about physical flexibility but about creating a ritual that signals the body and mind that it's time to wind down.

Soundscapes possess a profound impact on our ability to relax and drift into sleep. Whether it's the rhythmic whisper of white noise, the gentle patter of rain, or the soft cadences of ambient music, sound can act as a vehicle for relaxation. By incorporating these auditory elements into the sleep environment, individuals can create an auditory backdrop that masks disruptive noises and fosters a tranquil setting for sleep. This approach, supported by sound machines or apps designed for sleep, can be particularly effective for those whose minds are prone to nighttime wandering, offering a gentle, consistent stimulus to focus on while falling asleep.

Progressive muscle relaxation (PMR) is a technique that involves tensing and then relaxing each muscle group in the body, promoting physical and mental relaxation. Starting from the toes and moving upwards, this practice not only highlights areas of tension we may not be aware of but also teaches the body the contrast between tension and relaxation. By engaging in PMR in the evening, individuals can alleviate physical stress, signaling to the body that it's time to rest and recover. This method is especially beneficial for those who carry their stress physically, offering a direct route to relaxation and improved sleep quality.

The act of reflecting on positive aspects of one's life, or practicing gratitude, can have a surprisingly soothing effect on the mind, steering it away from the stressors and anxieties that may hinder sleep. By jotting down a few things one is grateful for each night, individuals can shift their focus from worry to well-being, fostering a positive mental environment conducive to sleep. This practice not only improves sleep quality by reducing the time it takes to fall asleep but also enhances the depth of sleep, contributing to a more restorative rest.

The culmination of these techniques forms a personalized sleep ritual, a series of steps tailored to the individual's unique needs and preferences that signal the transition from wakefulness to sleep. This ritual could involve a specific sequence of activities, such as a warm bath, reading by soft light, or listening to a guided meditation, all designed to cultivate a state of relaxation. By adhering to this ritual consistently, individuals can strengthen their body's response to these cues, further enhancing their ability to fall asleep and enjoy uninterrupted, quality rest.

In weaving these strands together—mindfulness, yoga, sound, muscle relaxation, and gratitude—individuals can construct a comprehensive approach to relaxation, tackling the barriers to sleep from multiple angles. This multifaceted strategy does not just address the symptoms of poor sleep but gets to the heart of the issue, fostering a deep, enduring change in sleep quality and, by extension, in overall health and well-being.

Lifelong Strategies for Health

Adapting Your Intermittent Diet Over Time

Intermittent fasting, a pattern of eating that cycles between periods of fasting and eating, has gained popularity as a method for weight loss, improved metabolic health, and increased longevity. However, as with any lifestyle change, the key to sustained success lies in the ability to adapt and evolve this approach over time. Life is not static; it is a dynamic journey marked by various physiological changes, lifestyle shifts, and evolving health goals. Therefore, your approach to intermittent fasting should be equally dynamic, reflecting the changing needs of your body and your life.

At the outset, it's crucial to recognize that the body's nutritional needs, metabolism, and response to fasting can change due to aging, hormonal shifts, activity levels, and health status. What works for you in your 30s may not suit your needs in your 50s and beyond. For instance, as metabolism naturally slows with age, the body's ability to recover from prolonged fasting periods might diminish, necessitating adjustments to your fasting regimen to maintain energy levels and nutritional balance.

The cornerstone of adapting your intermittent fasting approach is developing a keen awareness of your body's signals. Changes in energy levels, mood, sleep quality, and hunger cues can all indicate whether your current fasting schedule continues to serve your well-being or if adjustments are needed. Regular check-ins with a healthcare provider can offer insights into how your fasting regimen is affecting your overall health, including key markers such as blood sugar levels, cholesterol, and blood pressure.

One of the most powerful aspects of intermittent fasting is its inherent flexibility. There are several methods of intermittent fasting, ranging from the 16/8 method, where you fast for 16 hours and eat during an 8-hour window, to the 5:2 method, involving eating normally five days a week and reducing calorie intake on the other two days. As your life circumstances and health needs evolve, so too can your fasting schedule. For example, during periods of high stress or illness, shortening your fasting window or incorporating more nourishing, calorie-dense foods during your eating periods can help support your body's increased nutritional demands.

While intermittent fasting primarily focuses on when you eat, what you eat remains paramount. Adapting your diet to include a wide variety of nutrient-dense foods can help ensure that you're meeting your body's changing nutritional needs, even within restricted eating windows. As you age, prioritizing foods rich in calcium, vitamin D, fiber, and omega-3 fatty acids can support bone health, digestive wellness, and cardiovascular health, respectively. Moreover, incorporating more plant-based foods and lean proteins can support weight management and reduce the risk of chronic diseases.

Adapting your intermittent fasting approach over time isn't solely about adjusting your eating and fasting windows; it's also about integrating complementary lifestyle practices that support your overall health. Regular physical activity, whether it's walking, yoga, strength training, or any movement that you enjoy, can enhance the health benefits of intermittent fasting, including improving insulin sensitivity and supporting healthy weight management. Similarly, mindfulness practices like meditation and deep breathing can help manage the stress that may otherwise undermine your fasting efforts and overall health.

Ultimately, adapting your intermittent fasting diet over time is about embracing a holistic view of health—one that acknowledges the interconnectedness of diet, physical activity, mental well-being, and social connections. As you navigate through life's stages, your approach to fasting, like any aspect of your lifestyle, should be fluid, responsive to your body's needs, and reflective of your evolving goals for health and happiness.

In conclusion, the journey of intermittent fasting is one of personal discovery and adaptation. It's a practice that invites you to listen closely to your body, respond with compassion and flexibility, and continually seek a balance that nourishes you wholly—body, mind, and spirit. By remaining open to change and attentive to your evolving needs, intermittent fasting can be a valuable and sustainable component of a lifelong strategy for health and well-being.

Staying Engaged and Motivated

At the core of sustained motivation is a clear understanding of your 'why.' This encompasses more than the superficial goals of weight loss or fitness achievements; it's about connecting with the deeper reasons for choosing a healthier lifestyle. Whether it's the desire to be active and energetic for your children, to manage a chronic health condition, or simply to feel more vibrant and alive, anchoring to your why provides a reservoir of motivation that you can draw from when the going gets tough.

Goal setting is a powerful tool in maintaining motivation, but the efficacy of this tool lies in the nature of the goals set. Realistic, achievable, and time-bound goals that offer a sense of progress and achievement can reinforce motivation. Equally important is setting goals that are meaningful to you personally, which resonate with your values and aspirations. This could mean setting a goal to complete a 5K run, mastering a new cooking technique every month, or achieving a specific health marker like improved blood sugar levels.

Humans are inherently social beings, and the journey towards health is one that can be enriched and sustained by the support of a community. Engaging with others who share your goals and challenges can provide a sense of belonging, encouragement, and accountability. This community can be found in online forums, local fitness or nutrition groups, or among friends and family. Sharing experiences, celebrating each other's successes, and offering support during setbacks can amplify motivation and engagement.

Setbacks are an inevitable part of any long-term health journey. The key to maintaining motivation in the face of these challenges is resilience—the ability to bounce back and continue moving forward. This involves cultivating a mindset that views setbacks not as failures but as opportunities for learning and growth. It means forgiving yourself for lapses, understanding what led to them, and developing strategies to overcome similar challenges in the future.

Rigidity is the enemy of sustained motivation. Life's unpredictable nature means that the ability to adapt your health practices, including your approach to intermittent fasting, to changing circumstances is crucial for long-term success. This might mean adjusting your fasting windows, experimenting with different dietary approaches, or finding new ways to incorporate movement into your day. Mindfulness—being present and engaged with your experiences—can enhance your ability to listen to your body's needs and respond with kindness and flexibility.

Finally, maintaining motivation is about recognizing and

celebrating progress, no matter how small. Each step forward is a victory worth acknowledging. Practicing gratitude for what your body can do, for the nourishment you provide it, and for the moments of joy and satisfaction you experience along the way can fuel your motivation and commitment to your health journey.

In conclusion, staying engaged and motivated in your health journey, particularly when practicing intermittent fasting, is a multifaceted endeavor. It requires a deep connection to your personal why, setting realistic and meaningful goals, seeking support, learning from setbacks, embracing flexibility, and celebrating every step of progress. This holistic approach not only enhances your ability to maintain motivation but also enriches your journey towards health and well-being, making it a fulfilling and sustainable part of your life.

Planning for Success in All Areas of Life

1. Holistic Health Perspective

Adopting intermittent fasting is not just about diet manipulation; it's a lifestyle choice that impacts and is impacted by every aspect of your life. Recognizing that health is not merely the absence of disease but a state of complete physical, mental, and social well-being, it's crucial to approach IF with a holistic health perspective. This means acknowledging how your diet interacts with other areas of your life, including stress levels, sleep quality, physical activity, and emotional well-being.

2. Personalized Approach

Success in integrating IF into your life requires a personalized approach. Understand that there is no one-size-fits-all strategy. Pay attention to how your body and mind respond to different fasting schedules and adjust accordingly. Consider your daily routine, work demands, family responsibilities, and social life to tailor your IF approach in a way that feels sustainable and rewarding.

3. Balanced Nutrition

While IF focuses on when to eat, what you eat remains a cornerstone of your health. Planning for success involves preparing meals that are not only compatible with your fasting schedule but also nutritionally balanced. Emphasize whole foods, lean proteins, healthy fats, and a variety of fruits and vegetables to ensure your body receives the nutrients it needs to thrive.

4. Physical Activity

Regular physical activity complements intermittent fasting by enhancing metabolic health, improving mood, and supporting weight management. Incorporate activities you enjoy into your routine, whether it's walking, cycling, yoga, or weight training, to ensure consistency and enjoyment in your fitness journey.

5. Stress Management and Mental Health

Chronic stress and neglected mental health can undermine the benefits of IF by impacting your eating patterns, sleep quality, and overall well-being. Incorporate stress-reduction techniques such as meditation, deep breathing exercises, or mindfulness practices into your daily routine. Additionally, engaging in hobbies and activities that bring you joy can significantly contribute to your mental and emotional health.

6. Quality Sleep

As outlined in the previous sections, sleep plays a pivotal role in weight management and overall health. Prioritize sleep by establishing a consistent sleep schedule, creating a restful sleep environment, and adopting pre-sleep relaxation practices to enhance sleep quality. Remember, good sleep supports your body's recovery and is essential for the success of your IF journey.

7. Continuous Learning and Adaptation

The journey of health and wellness is one of continuous learning and adaptation. Stay informed about the latest research and developments in nutrition, intermittent fasting, and general health. Be open to experimenting with and adjusting your approach as you gain insights into what works best for your body and lifestyle.

8. Support System

Building a supportive community, whether online or in person, can provide encouragement, share knowledge, and offer accountability. Surround yourself with people who understand and support your health goals, and don't hesitate to seek professional guidance from healthcare providers, nutritionists, or fitness coaches when needed.

9. Reflection and Mindfulness

Regular reflection on your progress, challenges, and experiences can provide valuable insights into your health journey. Use journaling or mindfulness practices to connect with yourself, celebrate your achievements, and navigate challenges with compassion and resilience.

10. Integrating Joy and Flexibility

Lastly, ensure that your approach to health and intermittent fasting includes space for joy, flexibility, and indulgence in moderation. Allowing yourself occasional treats or adjustments to your fasting schedule for special occasions can make your health journey more enjoyable and sustainable.

Conclusion

Celebrating Your Journey

Embarking on a journey of health and wellness, particularly one that involves a significant lifestyle shift like intermittent fasting, is akin to setting sail on uncharted waters. It's a voyage that promises not only the discovery of new horizons but also encounters with storms and calm alike. Each milestone reached and every challenge overcome is a testament to your resilience, commitment, and growth. Celebrating your journey is not merely a matter of acknowledging achievements but embracing the entirety of your experience, with all its highs and lows, as a cohesive tapestry woven from your efforts, learnings, and transformations.

Celebration, in the context of your health journey, transcends the conventional festivities. It's an acknowledgment of your perseverance, a recognition of the strength you've mustered, and the challenges you've navigated. It's about honoring the commitment you made to yourself the moment you decided to take control of your health and well-being. This celebration is both a reflection on the path traversed and an affirmation of your ability to enact change in your life.

While milestones such as weight loss or fitness achievements often serve as tangible markers of progress, the essence of your journey encompasses much more. It includes the development of discipline, the deepening understanding of your body's needs, the cultivation of self-compassion, and the fostering of a mindful relationship with food and eating. Celebrating these intangible gains is equally, if not more, important, for they represent the foundational changes that ensure the sustainability of your wellness journey.

A pivotal component of celebration is reflection. Looking back on where you started, appreciating the effort you've invested, and acknowledging the growth you've experienced can be profoundly gratifying. It's also a practice in gratitude—not just for your achievements but for the learning opportunities your challenges presented. Reflecting on the moments of struggle and how you navigated them enriches your narrative, offering insights and strengths you carry forward.

Celebration is magnified when shared. Sharing your journey with others not only serves to inspire but also creates a space for communal support and encouragement. Your story could be the catalyst for someone else's beginning, a beacon of hope for those who may still be finding their way. Whether through social media, a blog, or casual conversations, opening up about your experiences contributes to a larger narrative of collective empowerment and wellness.

Incorporating rituals of celebration into your journey can enhance your sense of accomplishment and well-being. This could take many forms, from a quiet moment of meditation, acknowledging your progress, to more overt celebrations like a special meal, a new experience, or a physical token that symbolizes your achievement. These rituals, personalized to reflect what is most meaningful to you, act as milestones that punctuate your journey with joy and recognition.

Ultimately, celebrating your journey means embracing every part of it—the successes and the setbacks, the clarity and the confusion. It's about understanding that every step, whether forward or backward, is a part of the learning and growth process. This holistic embrace encourages a kinder, more compassionate approach to personal health and wellness goals, recognizing that perfection is not the aim but progress.

In conclusion, the journey of health and wellness, with intermittent fasting as one of its strategies, is a deeply personal and transformative experience. Celebrating this journey in all its facets not only honors the work you've done but also solidifies the foundation for continued growth, exploration, and well-being. It's a testament to the strength of the human spirit, the capacity for change, and the endless potential for renewal. Celebrating your journey is, in essence, celebrating yourself and the incredible capacity you have to shape your life and health for the better.

Embracing the Future with Confidence

From Uncertainty to Empowerment

The initial steps into intermittent fasting and lifestyle change are often marked by uncertainty and skepticism. However, as you navigate through the ebbs and flows of adapting to a new way of living, each challenge surmounted and each milestone achieved serves to transform uncertainty into a solid foundation of self-belief and empowerment. This journey teaches the invaluable lesson that change, while daunting, is both possible and rewarding. Carrying this empowerment forward, you stand ready to face future challenges not as insurmountable obstacles but as opportunities for further growth and self-discovery.

The Wisdom of Flexibility and Adaptation

Throughout your journey, one of the most critical lessons learned is the power of flexibility and adaptation. Just as you've adjusted your fasting schedules, dietary choices, and exercise routines in response to your body's needs and life's demands, this adaptability becomes a cornerstone of how you approach future goals. Life, in its essence, is unpredictable. The confidence to adapt and pivot when faced with new challenges or when pursuing new aspirations ensures that you are not rigidly bound to a single path but are open to exploring multiple avenues towards success and fulfillment.

The Strength of a Supportive Community

No journey of transformation is a solitary endeavor. Along the way, the value of a supportive community—be it family, friends, or fellow fasting practitioners—becomes abundantly clear. This network of support not only bolsters you through the challenging times but also celebrates your successes, big and small. As you look towards the future, the confidence to forge new connections and nurture existing ones underscores the strength derived from community. It's a reminder that while individual effort is paramount, shared experiences and support amplify resilience and confidence.

Grounded in Knowledge and Continuous Learning

Knowledge is a powerful ally on any journey of health and well-being. Your path has likely been punctuated with moments of learning—about nutrition, about your body's cues, about the science behind fasting. This pursuit of knowledge doesn't end with the achievement of your current goals. Instead, it opens up a landscape of continuous learning and curiosity. Embracing the future with confidence means carrying forward this thirst for knowledge, understanding that growth is an ongoing process, and what you know today is just the foundation for what you will learn tomorrow.

The Harmony of Mind, Body, and Spirit

Perhaps one of the most profound realizations on your journey is the interconnectedness of mind, body, and spirit. Wellness is not merely the absence of illness or the attainment of a certain physical aesthetic but a harmonious state where mental, physical, and emotional health are in alignment. This holistic approach to health, cultivated through your journey, provides a blueprint for facing the future. It ensures that your decisions, goals, and aspirations are not just focused on one aspect of well-being but encompass a balanced view of what it means to truly thrive.

Embracing the Unknown with Optimism

Finally, the journey through intermittent fasting and beyond teaches you to view the unknown not with fear but with optimism. Each step into the unfamiliar has built a resilience and a confidence that what lies ahead is not to be feared but embraced as part of the evolving journey of life. With the tools, knowledge, and experiences you've gathered, the future is a landscape ripe with potential, waiting to be explored with confidence and an open heart. In sum, embracing the future with confidence after a journey of health and transformation through intermittent fasting is about more than the goals achieved; it's about the person you've become in the process. It's a testament to the power of resilience, the importance of adaptability, the strength of community, the pursuit of knowledge, and the balance of holistic well-being. Armed with these insights and experiences, the path ahead is not just one to be walked but to be embraced with confidence, curiosity, and an unwavering belief in your ability to navigate whatever may come.

MEAL PLAN 30 DAYS

Week 1

Day of the Week	Breakfast	Lunch	Dinner
Monday	Greek yogurt with mixed berries	Grilled chicken salad with mixed greens	Baked salmon with steamed broccoli
Tuesday	Spinach and feta omelet with toast	Quinoa and black bean stuffed peppers	Chicken stir-fry with assorted vegetables
Wednesday	Smoothie with spinach, banana, and protein powder	Turkey and avocado wrap	Vegetable curry with brown rice
Thursday	Whole grain toast with avocado and poached egg	Salmon salad with mixed greens and vinaigrette	Grilled shrimp with quinoa salad
Friday	Cottage cheese with sliced peaches	Vegetable and hummus wrap	Beef and vegetable stew
Saturday	Oatmeal with almond butter and banana	Chicken Caesar salad	Pasta with marinara sauce and grilled vegetables
Sunday	Scrambled eggs with spinach and whole grain toast	Lentil soup with whole grain bread	Grilled chicken with asparagus and quinoa

Week 2

Day of the Week	Breakfast	Lunch	Dinner
Monday	Almond butter on whole grain toast	Spinach and quinoa salad with feta cheese	Lemon garlic tilapia with sautéed kale
Tuesday	Berry and banana smoothie with flaxseeds	Chicken avocado salad	Quinoa stuffed bell peppers
Wednesday	Poached eggs with asparagus on rye bread	Lentil and vegetable stew	Baked chicken breast with roasted vegetables
Thursday	Greek yogurt with granola and honey	Tuna salad on whole grain bread	Stir-fried tofu with broccoli and brown rice
Friday	Omelet with mushrooms, tomatoes, and onions	Beetroot and goat cheese arugula salad	Grilled salmon with sweet potato fries
Saturday	Pancakes with fresh strawberries and whipped cream	Turkey and cranberry sauce sandwich	Vegetable lasagna
Sunday	Avocado and egg breakfast sandwich	Soup of the day with a side of whole grain bread	Slow-cooked beef stew with root vegetables

Week 3

Day of the Week	Breakfast	Lunch	Dinner
Monday	Chia seed pudding with coconut milk and mango	Roasted vegetable and quinoa salad	Grilled trout with lemon butter and steamed green beans
Tuesday	Whole grain waffles with blueberries and yogurt	Mediterranean chickpea and cucumber salad	Spaghetti with marinara sauce and turkey meatballs
Wednesday	Avocado smoothie with spinach and protein powder	Tofu and vegetable stir-fry with rice	Roast chicken with carrots and potatoes
Thursday	Cottage cheese with pineapple	Turkey breast and avocado wrap	Fish tacos with cabbage slaw
Friday	Scrambled tofu with tomatoes and spinach	Salmon and avocado salad	Vegetarian chili with cornbread
Saturday	French toast with apple compote and cinnamon	Chicken orzo soup	Beef sirloin with roasted Brussels sprouts and quinoa
Sunday	Breakfast burrito with scrambled eggs, black beans, and salsa	Caprese salad with balsamic glaze	Baked cod with sweet potato mash and asparagus

Week 4

Day of the Week	Breakfast	Lunch	Dinner
Monday	Pear and walnut oatmeal	Grilled chicken Caesar salad	Pan-seared salmon with wild rice and asparagus
Tuesday	Protein smoothie with kale, banana, and almond milk	Beef and barley soup	Vegetarian moussaka
Wednesday	Avocado toast with cherry tomatoes	Shrimp and avocado salad	Chicken parmesan with spaghetti squash
Thursday	Quinoa breakfast bowl with fruits and nuts	Lentil salad with roasted vegetables	Pork tenderloin with apple sauce and green beans
Friday	Banana and peanut butter smoothie	Caprese stuffed avocado	Moroccan lamb stew with couscous
Saturday	Egg muffins with spinach and feta	Quinoa tabbouleh	Grilled vegetable kebabs with tzatziki sauce
Sunday	Granola with yogurt and mixed berries	Broccoli and cheddar soup	Roast beef with roasted root vegetables

Measurement Conversion Table

Volume Conversions

Volume (Liquid)	US Customary Units	Metric Units
1 teaspoon	1 tsp	5 milliliters (ml)
1 tablespoon	1 tbsp	15 milliliters
1 fluid ounce	1 fl oz	30 milliliters
1 cup	1 cup	240 milliliters
1 pint	1 pt	473 milliliters
1 quart	1 qt	946 milliliters
1 gallon	1 gal	3.785 liters

Weight Conversions

Weight	US Customary Units	Metric Units
1 ounce	1 oz	28 grams (g)
1 pound	1 lb	454 grams
1 kilogram	2.2 lbs	1000 grams (1 kg)

Length Conversions

Length	US Customary Units	Metric Units

		2.54 centimeters (cm)
1 inch	1 in	
1 foot	1 ft	30.48 centimeters

Metric Volume Conversions

Volume	Metric Units	US Customary Units
1 milliliter (ml)	1 ml	0.034 fluid ounce (fl oz)
100 milliliters	100 ml	3.4 fluid ounces
1 liter (L)	1 L	34 fluid ounces
		4.2 cups
		2.1 pints
		1.06 quarts
		0.26 gallon

Metric Weight Conversions

Weight	Metric Units	US Customary Units
1 gram (g)	1 g	0.035 ounces (oz)
100 grams	100 g	3.5 ounces
500 grams	500 g	1.1 pounds (lb)
1 kilogram (kg)	1 kg	2.2 pounds

Temperature Conversions

Temperature	Celsius (°C)	Fahrenheit (°F)
Freezing Point	0°C	32°F
Refrigerator	4°C	39°F
Room Temperature	20°C - 22°C	68°F - 72°F
Boiling Water	100°C	212°F